"*Feed your Fertility* provides solid information and advice on the most fundamental strategy for increased fertility. We have developed much in the way of high technology, but the foods we eat every day are our most powerful medicine. Laura and Emily provide a path to nourishing yourself not in only body, but in mind and spirit as well."

—Chris Axelrad, L.Ac., FABORM, president of the
American Board of Oriental Reproductive Medicine

"*Feed Your Fertility* is a wonderful and refreshing multifaceted approach towards reproductive care. From diet to stress reduction to conventional fertility treatments and Eastern methodologies, this book is a comprehensive guide for fertility care and successful, healthy pregnancies."

—Eliran Mor, M.D., California Center for Reproductive Health

"*Feed Your Fertility* is a must-read for anyone trying to conceive. It draws on traditional Chinese medicine brought right up-to-date, offering couples a simple but effective nutritional plan that works. I recommend it highly."

—Jill Blakeway, M.S., L.Ac., co-author,
Making Babies: A Proven 3-Month Program for Maximum Fertility

"[This book] is a must for anyone who wants to optimize their success by integrating Eastern and Western medicine. It is a comprehensive resource outlining a mind–body evaluation and approach to fertility."

—Kelly J. Baek, M.D., California Fertility Partners

"*Feed Your Fertility* is really an invitation to pursue the best that life has to offer: the beauty of Earth's bounty, refining and cultivating your own intuition, sharing this wisdom with your loved ones, and passing along the delicious truth to your children. Food is our medicine, and thus the holistic circle ripples and expands."

—Lilakoi Moon (formerly Lisa Bonet), actress and mother

"If you're caught in a quagmire of conflicting information about infertility, its causes, and its treatment, you need this book. Accessible and easy to read, it's a wealth of information that addresses everything from environmental toxins, diet, and Chinese medicine to PCOS, endometriosis, and standard medical fertility treatments. Emily and Laura approach these issues with wisdom, kindness, and a firm can-do attitude that will help you conquer stress AND beat back your infertility!"

—Kristen Michaelis, author of *Beautiful Babies: Nutrition for Fertility,*
Pregnancy, Breastfeeding, and Baby's First Foods

"*Feed Your Fertility* is a wonderful reminder of not only the mind–body connection, but the connection between ourselves and our environment and how they both affect our health and ability to conceive. The knowledge you will gather from this book will give you the power to cultivate a healthy lifestyle, body, and pregnancy."

—Jill Latiano Howerton, executive producer of the film *GMO OMG*

To our children—
Will, Sebastian, and Frankie—and all future
generations. May you enjoy a fertile world.

First published in the USA in 2015 by
Fair Winds Press, a member of
Quarto Publishing Group USA Inc.
100 Cummings Center
Suite 406-L
Beverly, MA 01915-6101
www.fairwindspress.com
Visit www.bodymindbeautyhealth.com. It's your personal guide to a
happy, healthy, and extraordinary life!

19 18 17 16 15   1 2 3 4 5

ISBN: 978-1-59233-662-3

Digital edition published in 2015
eISBN: 978-1-62788-285-9

Library of Congress Cataloging-in-Publication Data available

Cover and book design by Rita Sowins / Sowins Design
Cover images courtesy of Shutterstock.com; bottom left image courtesy
     of the authors
Printed and bound in the United States

*The information in this book is for educational purposes only. It is not
intended to replace the advice of a physician or medical practitioner. Please
see your health care provider before beginning any new health program.*

Feed Your Fertility

**Your Guide to Cultivating a Healthy Pregnancy with
Traditional Chinese Medicine, Real Food, and Holistic Living**

Emily Bartlett, LAc &
Laura Erlich, LAc

Fair Winds Press
100 Cummings Center, Suite 406L
Beverly, MA 01915

fairwindspress.com • bodymindbeautyhealth.com

Contents

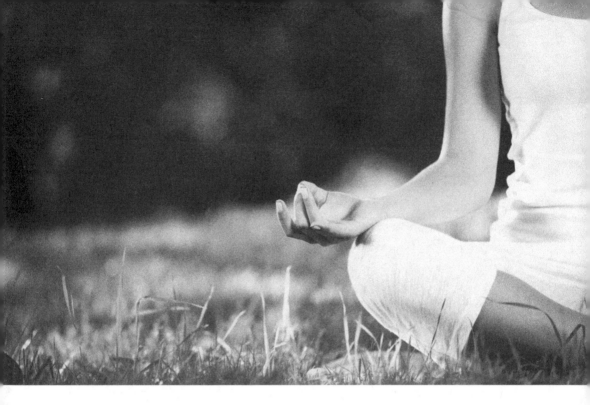

Introduction

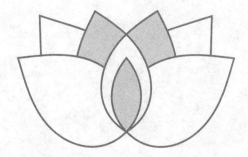

WHILE THE DECISION TO START A FAMILY can be both exciting and terrifying, it is especially so for couples who encounter challenges. At its best, making a baby can be the thrill and joy of a lifetime. At its worst, it can be a roller coaster of hope, disappointment, and unfulfilled dreams.

We wrote this book to take the chaos and confusion down a notch and put you back in the driver's seat. Is your diet nourishing you and contributing to your ability to conceive? Have you explored the unique perspectives on fertility that Chinese medicine can provide? Are you getting the most out of your medical care? Have you *truly* created space in your life for a new little being?

The title we chose, *Feed Your Fertility*, has to do with a lot more than food. We believe that, in order to truly nourish yourself in a meaningful way, all aspects of your life must be fed. That means paying attention to your relationships, your lifestyle habits, and all of the nuances that go into making you feel healthy, inside and out. In this book, we hope to provide you with tools to enhance your whole self, paving the way toward conception, a healthy pregnancy, and a thriving baby.

Taking this a leap further, in Chinese medicine, human beings (and all living beings) are viewed as a microcosm of the world in which we live. This means that we as individuals are simply tiny parts of the greater whole, and our little tiny part is a mirror image of the world around us, just on a much smaller scale.

With this in mind, we admit that this book is about more than achieving a healthy pregnancy—it's a call to cultivate fertility within your life and for our planet at large. Without an external healthy environment, our internal environments become essentially irrelevant, because we cannot survive without the earth upon which we live. By living consciously and choosing our food sources carefully, we take on the role of the archetypal Mother, nourishing ourselves, the health of our planet, and the viability of future generations.

As part of your fertility journey, we invite you to embrace the role of the great archetypal Mother, bestowed with the obligation to protect her children. Begin to live your life from the belief that you already are a mother and that your mothering can be applied right here and now.

Consider the possibility of letting go of the wanting and instead living through the present moment—honoring, cultivating, and activating life and fertility in every aspect of your existence. Living from this place, on both a physical and energetic level, will invite the conception of a baby into your body far more readily than existing from a state of fear, stress, and ticking clocks.

Emily   Laura

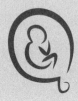

PART 1

Causes of Infertility

Prospective parents, it's time to get healthy. Now's your chance to finally quit smoking, stop binge drinking, and stop depending on sleep medications, caffeine, and other chemicals you can do without. Start exercising, see a therapist to get over your issues with your mother-in-law, stop overworking, and start eating healthy foods from sustainable sources. Sounds simple, right?

Even if you don't feel like you have any major issues to overcome, there still may be barriers standing in your way to conception including mounting stress, a myriad of hidden toxins, and the pitfalls of our broken food system.

Chapter 1

Stress, the Baby Blocker

ASIDE FROM POOR DIET, stress is the biggest contributor to modern health problems. The truth is that stress is unavoidable. It's as integral to being human as eating and sleeping. In fact, our very survival depends on our ability to react to our surroundings via our stress mechanisms.

Have you heard of "fight-or-flight?" This is the part of your nervous system (called the sympathetic nervous system) that, when activated, will give you superhuman powers for survival by sending extra blood flow to your muscles, making your vision more acute, and sharpening your reflexes. The sympathetic nervous system can ask the body to perform out-of-the-ordinary feats because it temporarily deprioritizes normal body function, including digestion, sleep, and . . . reproduction. After all, why would your body agree to make a baby if there was a pretty good chance your life was in acute danger?

In our modern hustle-bustle, go-go-go world, it's common for your nervous system to always be in a state of mild to moderate fight-or-flight, telling your reproductive system to take a nap. Recent research supports the theory that stress negatively impacts fertility. Researchers at Columbia University published a 2014 study in *Fertility and Sterility*, that concluded that stress diminishes male sperm count and motility. Another 2014 study published in *Human Reproduction* found that women with elevated salivary alpha-amylase (a marker of chronic elevated stress) had more than double the risk of infertility. Studies aside, common sense suggests that by reducing and managing your stress, you may increase your likelihood of conception by improving your overall health.

Here's another simple fact: Baby-making itself can be stressful, especially when months tick by without getting pregnant. What's more, the stress of trying to conceive can often drain the fun and enjoyment out of sex, leading to strain in your relationship.

If all of this news seems rather, well, stressful—don't fret. In Part 2 (page 34), we will be arming you with a myriad of ways to manage and deactivate your stress. First, let's look at some other silent fertility offenders that can be found in places you may least expect.

Chapter 2

Toxins, Toxins Everywhere

SHORT OF MOVING TO THE WILDERNESS WITHOUT A CAR, you can't completely eliminate environmental toxins, but you can use common sense to avoid excessive exposure in everything from the water you drink to lubrication you may use in the bedroom.

∼ Understanding Xenoestrogens ∽

For starters, we need to talk about xenoestrogens because they have the potential to have a direct effect on your fertility, your health, and your future offspring. Xenoestrogens are chemical compounds that imitate estrogen in the body. They can be either naturally occurring or synthetic.

Natural xenoestrogens come primarily from plants (often called phytoestrogens), and we mostly get exposed to them through food such as soy. Synthetic xenoestrogens are extremely prevalent in our environment and include things such as PCBs (in insulation and oil-based paints), BPA (in plastic), and phthalates (in cosmetics, lubricants, food packaging, and more).

Xenoestrogens are a problem because they act as endocrine disruptors, basically filling the receptors for true estrogen in the body, which is an issue whether you're starting with too much, too little, or just the right amount of this hormone in the first place. The resulting hormone imbalance directly interferes with reproductive health and has also been associated with early puberty in both boys and girls.

Here are some guidelines to minimize your xenoestrogen exposure:

* **DO NOT DRINK FROM PLASTIC WATER BOTTLES** that have been heated up by the sun or sitting in a hot car. It's best not to reuse plastic water bottles—glass or stainless steel is optimal.

* **AVOID TOO MUCH CHLORINE EXPOSURE** by buying chlorine-free paper products, including tampons, menstrual pads, and household paper products. Be sure to rinse well before and after swimming in a chlorinated pool.
* **SWITCH TO NONTOXIC HOUSEHOLD CLEANERS, TOILETRIES, AND COSMETICS.** Bleach, ammonia, and other chemicals found in household cleaners are toxic and should be removed from your home. Nontoxic alternatives are available—from window cleaner to dish and laundry soap. There are also lots of easy DIY recipes out there that are both easy to make and easy on your wallet.
* **BUY ORGANIC** produce, meats, and dairy products to avoid pesticides and hormones.
* **STORE YOUR FOOD IN GLASS CONTAINERS;** avoid plastic as much as possible, and definitely do not microwave or bake food in plastic.
* **IF YOU'VE BEEN A SMOKER OF ANY SUBSTANCE, WE'RE GOING TO ASSUME THAT YOU'VE QUIT.** (If not, talk to your acupuncturist about a plan ASAP.) If your family or friends smoke, steer clear as much as possible, making sure that anyone you live with moves his or her habit to the patio at the very least.
* **IF YOU PAINT OR OTHERWISE WORK WITH TOXIC CHEMICALS, REDUCE YOUR EXPOSURE AS MUCH AS POSSIBLE,** and—in addition to your nutrient-dense diet—make sure to supplement with glutathione and other antioxidants discussed on page 144.
* **DITCH THE PERFUMES.** They may smell nice, but the chemicals in synthetic scents may disrupt your hormones. Avoid them in all forms—spray-ons, lotions, deodorants, air fresheners, etc. Essential oils make an excellent replacement.

∼ Filter Your Water ∼

All of the water that comes in contact with your body (both internal and external) should be filtered to remove chlorine, fluoride, and other toxic chemicals, due to the risk of exposure to xenoestrogens and other endocrine disruptors. There are many different and often confusing water filtration options out there. Here's a rundown:
* **BEST**—Whole house filter for bathing and for drinking and a separate reverse osmosis filter (and a method to add minerals back into the water either via a specialized filter or mineral drops that you can buy online or at a health food store)
* **GOOD**—A filter attached to the tap of your shower and/or bath plus reverse osmosis filter and minerals as above
* **NOT GOOD ENOUGH**—Brita filters, bathing in municipal tap water, reverse osmosis water without added minerals

～ Moderate Medications ～

For those who are trying to conceive naturally, the simple answer is to keep medication to a minimum. Many symptoms and health imbalances (such as difficulty sleeping, headaches, and anxiety) can be addressed as you work with your Chinese medicine practitioner.

OVER-THE-COUNTER PAIN MEDS

Ibuprofen, aspirin, and naproxen are in a class of pain-relieving drugs known as NSAIDs (short for nonsteroidal anti-inflammatory drugs). While these pills may seem like a quick fix for a headache or menstrual cramps, the pathway they block to eliminate pain is the same pathway used in the release of a mature egg at ovulation.

NSAIDs use can result in a type of ovulation failure called Luteinized Unruptured Follicle Syndrome (LUFTS), where the ovary matures a follicle, but the egg doesn't pop out in response to the signal to ovulate (the LH surge). Luckily, this condition is reversible once NSAID ingestion is stopped, but we still don't recommend using these medicines unless absolutely necessary.

ANTIDEPRESSANTS AND OTHER DRUGS TO REGULATE MOOD

The use of antidepressant and antianxiety medications remains controversial. Overall, medical professionals agree that depression in and of itself can be quite harmful to pregnancy, so measures should be taken to ensure that a pregnant woman is not suffering from clinical depression that may impede her ability to care for herself or her unborn child properly.

On the other hand, most antianxiety medicines are not advised during pregnancy because they affect the body in a way that may be altered by pregnancy hormones.

Whether you are trying to conceive or are already pregnant, it is essential to be under the care of a psychiatrist or psycho-pharmacologist who has expert knowledge of the use of these drugs during gestation and the postpartum period.

Finally, it's important to consider what has occurred in your life that made it necessary to start taking these medications in the first place. If you suffer from situational depression or anxiety, might it be possible to consider a step-down from your medication (under the care of your doctor, of course) now that you're expecting? If you are clinically depressed, regardless of what is happening in your life, coming off medication may not be for you. In either case, there are many natural and holistic alternatives you might consider (under the supervision of your medical and holistic care providers) to minimize your exposure and maximize your well-being during this sensitive time.

BIRTH CONTROL

Oral contraceptives are so common in our culture that everyone knows them as simply "the pill." Prescribed like candy by most OB-GYNs, most people don't realize that long-term use of those little baby blockers can have a negative impact on future fertility and overall health.

"The pill" (or the patch, ring, or shot—they all deliver the same medicine, for the most part) does not come without its problems, including the consequences of high estrogen, damaged gut flora, potential suppression of reproductive problems, and the obvious yet significant function of delaying baby-making.

Birth control pills work by tricking your body into suppressing ovulation by keeping your estrogen levels high. Estrogen dominance comes with a long list of side effects and health consequences, including reduced sex drive, weight gain, melasma (brown spots on the face), mood swings, and an increased risk of blood clotting, stroke, and breast cancer.

Hormone replacement therapy, including oral birth control, has a damaging effect on the bacteria in our intestines. The result of long-term exposure to these hormones is an overgrowth of the intestinal bacteria *Candida albicans*, which can lead to increased yeast infections and food sensitivities, as well as impaired immune function and nutrient absorption. Women who are (or were) on birth control should take measures to balance their gut flora, through probiotic supplementation and consuming plenty of probiotic-rich foods such as cultured veggies, kombucha tea, and kefir—a subject we will cover in much more detail in a later chapter.

Many women are prescribed the pill early in their reproductive life because of painful or irregular periods, acne, and mood swings. Often, the pill serves as a cover-up for more serious conditions, including PCOS and endometriosis. While no one wants to deal with the discomfort of these disorders, pushing them into latency until you are ready to have a baby is fraught with problems. We treat so many women well into their thirties and early forties who have been on birth control since they were teenagers. Discovering that you have been suppressing a condition that may require surgery or advanced medical intervention can throw a serious monkey wrench into baby-making plans.

Once the symbol of sexual liberation, birth control has played a powerful role in the postponement of starting a family. While we are all for a woman choosing her own destiny and having a child when she is ready, the mind-set that it is possible to wait as long as you want to make a baby is simply false. We feel that true equality will come when women are supported in having a family at an age when their fertility is most promising, without any punitive effects on their professional lives.

FERTILITY MEDICATION

When it comes to Western fertility treatments, some couples find themselves taking way more medication than they ever have in their lives as part of the process. From hormones to build your uterine lining and increase follicle counts, to suppressive drugs such as Lupron to prevent an early lead follicle, to ovarian stimulants such as Clomid and gonadotropins, to HCG shots and progesterone to encourage ovulation and support pregnancy—you may feel like a walking pharmacy. In these cases, do your best to go with the flow.

Acupuncture and Chinese herbs (when prescribed by an herbalist who specializes in reproductive health) can be quite helpful in moderating the negative effects of drugs, without getting in the way of their function and detoxing when the cycle is over and/or you are pregnant.

Sometimes, birth control pills are used in the short term as part of an IVF protocol. If those are your doctor's orders, please don't sweat it. Short bursts of ovarian suppression won't wreak havoc on your endocrine system the way that long-term use will.

✳ USE THE RIGHT LUBE ✳

If you need or prefer extra glide during sex, you may opt for using lubricants. Here's the problem: Most lubricants act as spermicides, even if they aren't advertised to kill sperm.

A woman's cervical fluid is a perfectly designed medium in which sperm swim to their target—the egg, so care must be taken in choosing additional lubricants.

While some natural-minded folks choose coconut oil or other oils for lubrication, it is unclear whether this is an ideal medium for sperm conduction. Luckily, you can use egg white as a sperm-friendly, natural lubricant right out of the fridge. For those looking for something less, um, culinary, there are several sperm-friendly lubricants on the market, such as Pre-Seed. (Though we *would* prefer if they would make this product paraben-free.)

Chapter 3

The Standard American Diet and Fertility—What Is Going Wrong?

AT THE RISK OF SOUNDING A FEW DECADES OLDER THAN WE ARE, food just isn't what it used to be. From new-fangled processed and fake foods to destructive farming methods and genetically modified organisms, when it comes to modern foods: buyer beware.

~ Processed Foods ~

Don't you find it weird that you can have milk for weeks and weeks in the fridge that doesn't go sour? If you don't, you should. The same goes for boxes of cereal or crackers that may get stale, but never really spoil. Even grocery store fruit lasts a freakishly long time on the countertop and sometimes never goes bad.

We're all for convenience, but as farmer and visionary extraordinaire Joel Salatin has titled his book, "*Folks, this ain't normal.*"

Additives and preservatives make it possible for food to never go bad. The issue here is that additives and preservatives are only sort-of safe to eat, creating immediate and long-term complications for our health. Another problem with food that doesn't go bad is that it's missing the living enzymes and beneficial microbes our bodies need.

No matter how busy you are, if you are trying to conceive, you should not be eating for convenience—you should be eating for fertility. Period. Every bite should count.

∾ Franken-Foods ∾

Fake foods are so omnipresent in our modern food supply that they largely go unnoticed. Just start reading labels in a conventional grocery store if you find this fact surprising. Sadly, through powerful lobbies in the food industry, franken-foods legally fly under our radar: imitation "cheese" food, juice that's packed with high-fructose corn syrup, margarine spread made with "healthy" industrial vegetable oils, chocolate that is mostly hydrogenated fats, and sweets that are tricking your brain with toxic chemicals. Yuck.

This excerpt from *In Defense of Food*, by Michael Pollan, provides some historical context for how fake foods have made their way snugly into our food system:

> *The 1938 Food, Drug, and Cosmetic Act imposed strict rules requiring that the word "imitation" appear on any food product that was, well, an imitation . . . The food industry [argued over the word], strenuously for decades, and in 1973 it finally succeeded in getting the imitation rule tossed out, a little-noticed but momentous step that helped speed America down the path of nutritionism.*

HERE'S A LIST OF INGREDIENTS TO LOOK OUT FOR AND ELIMINATE FROM YOUR DIET:

* "Foods" containing "vegetable oil," cottonseed oil (buh-bye fast-food french fries), soybean oil, shortening, margarine, corn oil, canola oil, sunflower oil, or any use of the word "hydrogenated"
* "Foods" with artificial sweeteners
* "Foods" that say "natural flavor" or "natural coloring," which are often duping you with fake petrochemical-based toxins
* Low fat "foods"—not only do you need the fat, but low-fat foods (including skim milk) tend to contain nonfat milk powder. You won't find this on the label because it's technically milk, but nonfat milk powder is a toxic substance containing oxidized cholesterol. In addition, low-fat products may contain guar gum, carrageenan, soy protein, cornstarch, or any kind of chemical compound a scientist can dream up.

The moral of the story: Buy organic and get familiar with the sources of your food.

∾ Organic and Seasonal versus Conventional Produce ∾

A study by Stanford University researchers published in the *Annals of Internal Medicine* examined 240 organic and nonorganic fruits, vegetables, grains, meat, poultry, eggs, and milk for nutrient and contaminant levels.

The researchers found that more than one-third of conventional produce had detectable pesticide residues, compared with 7 percent of organic produce samples. It also found organic meats were one-third less likely to carry bacteria resistant to antibiotics than conventionally produced meat.

Additionally, they found that organic foods, on the whole, don't contain any more vitamins or nutrients than conventional foods; going organic is less about what you're missing and more about the extra toxic load on your body when you don't choose organic.

Though not addressed within this study, another reason to go organic (or even better, grow your own fruits and veggies) is that shelf life is a dominant priority for grocery store produce. Because of this, even organic produce is often sprayed with bleach solution to kill any microorganisms on the surface, which accelerate the time it takes for the fruit to rot. While the bleach evaporates and the internal nutrition of the fruit is preserved, the fruit no longer bears the probiotic flora it did when plucked fresh off the tree or bush, bequeathing the eater (you) with nothing when it comes to healthy microflora.

By choosing organic, seasonal produce, you are eating foods appropriate for best nutrition during the current time of year. For example, watermelon in the summer is cooling and hydrating, and butternut squash in the autumn builds blood and supports digestive health for a long winter ahead. In many locales, citrus is in season in the winter when our immune systems can certainly use an antioxidant boost.

To ensure you're eating seasonal, local, and organic produce, visit your local farmers' markets or sign up for a CSA farm box. Eating with the seasons is not only good for your body and the earth but is good for your budget, too.

≈ The Problem with Conventional Meat Production ↩

The industrialized meat industry in the United States is what gives meat-eating a bad name. CAFOs (Concentrated Animal Feeding Operations) or IFAP (Industrial Farm Animal Production) are the factories that grow 99 percent of meat in America.

Cattle are herbivores, designed by nature to eat grass and clover (the fresher the better), while CAFOs cattle are fed genetically modified corn mixed with hay and industry by-products. Cows eating corn is a bit like humans eating Lucky Charms—for every meal. It's not good. Improper diet tends to create health problems for the animals, so they are often given antibiotics as a routine measure. They are crowded into grassless bits of land, so you have unhealthy, stressed-out cattle, standing in their own excrement.

Because of their poor diet and conditions, when meat from these cattle is processed, it needs to be uniformly decontaminated, so it's sprayed with ammonia. Yes, you read that right—*sprayed with ammonia.*

So besides the obvious pairing with potatoes fried in rancid vegetable oil, your Big Mac certainly has plenty of reasons to contribute to heart disease, cancer, and other ailments—including infertility. With 99 percent of meat coming from this type of operation, it is no wonder beef has developed such a bad reputation.

MEAT AND THE ENVIRONMENT

Many folks choose vegetarianism for moral and environmental reasons. Based on all of the problems with factory meat, this rationale makes perfect sense. Conventionally farmed meat, poultry, and dairy are not only detrimental to your body and inhumane to the animals, but these practices are also devastating to our environment.

In the American farm belt, the last several decades have been plagued with polluted groundwater, inert soil, acid rain, and sick animals—including nearly wiping out the bee population. These seemingly insignificant buzzing insects play a vital role in the agricultural ecosystem. Without bees to pollinate crops, we can expect food shortages and larger crises around the corner. While there are many causative and contributing factors to this ecological crisis, the use of fossil fuel–based fertilizers and toxic pesticides play a large role.

Most farmers' market–going, health-conscious folks know that choosing locally grown, organic fruits and veggies is a smart way to circumvent the mess of corporate agribusiness. This principle applies to meat, poultry, eggs, and dairy as well.

Unlike conventionally farmed meat, pasture-raised, sustainably farmed animals are actually *much better* for the environment. For starters, these animals are not reliant on toxic GMO corn crops as the cornerstone of their nutrition. Proper farming techniques can actually contribute to a *reduction* in carbon saturation in the atmosphere through crop rotation and properly fertilized farmlands, so by choosing pasture-raised beef, dairy, poultry, and eggs, you are actually reducing the load on planet earth. Don't worry—we won't make you hug trees next (unless you want to, of course).

Chinese medicine views the human body as a microcosm of the environment—meaning what happens on the outside will be mirrored by what happens within your body. Avoiding factory-raised meat (including meat served at most restaurants) is vitally important, for the fertility of your body as well as for the land.

～ Infertility and GMOs ～

For centuries, gardeners, farmers, and scientists have been crossbreeding plants and animals (within the same species) to create the most desired traits. Genetically modified organisms were first introduced into our food supply in 1994 and are created by the introduction of *foreign* genetic proteins from other species to change the way the plant or animal's genes express.

While in theory such an amazing biotechnology could be used to make plants more nutritious or able to grow in harsh climates thus solving the issues of world hunger, in reality, this is not happening. Monsanto and other megacorporations are using GMOs to create pesticide-tolerant, patented seed crops that do not last for more than one season. This creates dominance over small farmers who previously bought seeds only once and now must buy seeds every time they plant, along with the pesticides and herbicides these new varieties of crops require.

Besides the economical and ethical issues involved with GMO crops, it is very likely that the genetic alteration of food will have an impact on those animals and people that are consuming the food. How's this for freaky?

ONCE EATEN, GMOS MAY STAY INSIDE YOUR BODY FOREVER

The only published study on the effect of GMOs on the human body revealed what may be the most dangerous problem with genetically modified foods: the gene inserted into genetically modified soy transfers into the DNA of bacteria living inside our intestines and *continues* to function. This means that long after we stop eating GMOs, we may still have potentially harmful genetically modified proteins produced continuously inside of us. Put more plainly, eating corn chips produced from genetically modified corn might transform our intestinal bacteria into living pesticide factories, possibly for the rest of our lives.

When evidence of gene transfer is reported at medical conferences around the United States, doctors often respond by citing the huge increase of gastrointestinal problems among their patients over the last decade. Genetically modified foods may be colonizing the gut flora of North Americans—and not in any desirable way.

GMO FOODS ARE LADEN WITH CHEMICALS

Among scientists, it is still a hot debate whether or not GMOs are specifically the cause of infertility and other health issues.

Beyond the possibility that GMOs themselves are a problem, it cannot be denied that genetically modified foods such as "Roundup Ready Corn" are also engineered to withstand high exposure to pesticides and herbicides. Even if messing with genes in fruits and vegetables does NOT cause infertility, it is certain these poisons are wreaking havoc on our health—whether consumed directly, in or on fruits and vegetables, or via the meat of animals that have eaten GMO feed.

Glyphosate, one of the active ingredients in Roundup and other herbicides, is a known endocrine disruptor, meaning it interferes with hormone balance in the body and is able to induce health issues with even a small amount of exposure. Aside from infertility, endocrine disruptors can affect mood and metabolism and have been linked to some cancers as well. It is advised not only to avoid pesticide-laden foods, but also to filter your water, which may also be contaminated with glyphosate from agricultural runoff.

GMO FOODS OFFER INFERIOR NUTRITION

Finally, if franken-foods and poison sprays aren't enough, we need to talk about the whole point of food in the first place—nutrition. It's important to note that nutritional quality is not a priority when it comes to genetically modified produce: economic dominance, extended shelf life, herbicide resistance, and the ability to grow in crowded rows and in nutrient-deficient soil are the current goals of genetic modifications.

When it comes to making babies, what we eat is of utmost importance. Whether you are just starting to think about having a baby or are having problems trying to conceive, it is essential that you eat the most nutritious food possible. It's a no-brainer— eliminate GMOs from your diet if you want to make a healthy baby.

There have been various studies that link GMOs and infertility, which are contested feverishly by GMO supporters:

* A study of hamsters in Russia demonstrated nearly complete infertility after three generations were fed genetically modified soy. Any babies that were born suffered

from slow growth and high mortality rates. Alexey Surov, the biologist in charge of these studies, says, "We have no right to use GMOs until we understand the possible adverse effects, not only to ourselves but to future generations as well."

* Another study, conducted by Dr. Irina Ermakova of the Institute of Higher Nervous Activity and Neurophysiology in Moscow, a part of the Russian Academy of Sciences, showed that rats fed genetically modified soy died at a rate FIVE times higher than rats fed GMO-free soy. The babies in the group who consumed genetically modified soy were also smaller and could not reproduce. The male rats' testicles turned from a normal pink color to a purplish-blue when fed GMOs, and their sperm quality was poor.

* An Austrian government study published in November 2008 showed that the more genetically modified corn was fed to mice, the fewer babies they had and the smaller the babies were.

* According to the Institute for Responsible Technology, farmers in the United States and India have reported sterility and death of livestock after introducing genetically modified feed.

This is only a partial list of studies and reports. While no large-scale human clinical trials have been funded, doctors and other experts are recommending a GMO-free diet for various health conditions, including infertility.

HOW TO AVOID GMOS

Here are the top ways to steer clear of GMOs:

* **EAT ORGANIC**—The easiest way to avoid GMOs is to only eat 100 percent certified organic foods because the USDA requires that organic food be not genetically modified.

* **AVOID THE BIG GMO CROPS**—If you cannot afford 100 percent organic, be sure to avoid nonorganic foods that contain these ingredients: corn, soy, canola, and sugar (usually made from genetically modified sugar beets).

* **DON'T EAT PACKAGED FOODS**—Even packaged foods labeled "organic" may not contain all-organic, non-GMO ingredients. Packaged foods labeled "organic" can contain up to 5 percent nonorganic ingredients, including GMOs.

* **READ YOUR LABELS**—In an ideal world you won't be eating processed foods, but if you do, be sure to read your labels to look out for the major GMO products above.

* **KNOW YOUR FARMER**—The absolute best way to know what's in your food is to know exactly where it came from. While this may seem like an inconvenience to your life, we guarantee infertility or cancer are bigger inconveniences. So get out to your local farmers' market, ask questions, and find out how your food is grown.

While we're not usually apt to take health advice from a health insurance company, for once the corporate bottom line *does* line up with consumers' best interests. Skip GMOs, stay healthy, save everyone money—and increase fertility while you're at it.

∼ The Myths of Popular Fertility Diets ∼

In writing a book about fertility and food, we did our homework to see what the other experts are recommending. Just about everyone can agree that processed, packaged foods are not a good idea when you're trying to conceive, but beyond that, we were shocked to find a startling collection of myths from one book to the next.

FERTILITY FOOD MYTH #1: AVOID SATURATED FAT AND EAT ONLY "HEALTHY FATS" (OR LOW-FAT)

While most people know that monounsaturated fats are good and trans fats are bad, you may be surprised to read that saturated fat and cholesterol are actually good for you, and the new-fangled, so-called "heart-healthy" fats are not.

Yep, you read correctly—saturated fat and cholesterol are essential to human health. Despite the common misconceptions and bad reputation it has undeservedly earned, saturated fat doesn't clog arteries or cause heart disease. Saturated fat *does* support most of the body's critical functions including a healthy brain and nervous system, strong bones and teeth, optimal lung capacity, and healthy hormone function.

Including them liberally in your diet will help to optimize your baby-making potential and ensure the health of your child.

When you consider that humans have been thriving on diets rich in saturated fat for millions of years, it just doesn't make logical sense that it could be so unhealthy. It turns out that the consumption of industrial polyunsaturated fats is the single most prevalent change to our diet in recent history. Compared to one hundred years ago, modern humans eat about the same amount of carbohydrates, protein, and saturated fat, but over *two-and-a-half times* the amount of polyunsaturated fat. Simultaneously the rates of heart disease, obesity, and diabetes have also climbed.

THE DANGERS OF CANOLA OIL

Because of its stable chemical structure, saturated fat is far safer for cooking than new-fangled cooking oils such as corn, sunflower, and vegetable a.k.a. soybean, grape seed, cottonseed AND canola oils. These nontraditional vegetable oils are packed with PUFAs. What's a PUFA? We're so glad you asked.

PUFA stands for polyunsaturated fatty acids. Whereas saturated fatty acids are made stable with hydrogen atoms, *unsaturated* fatty acids have incomplete bonds on each link of their chain, making each of their multiple (poly) bonds very unstable and prone to oxidation.

The volatile nature of PUFA is why they are dangerous to your body. It's really pretty simple. PUFAs are bad; saturated fat is rad.

···
FERTILITY FOOD MYTH #2: FOCUS ON LEAN MEATS AND REDUCE MEAT CONSUMPTION
···

Many of the popular recommendations for fertility diets encourage hopeful couples to reduce meat consumption and focus on lean meats. Because saturated fat and cholesterol (from healthy animal sources) are *essential* to hormone health and fertility—this recommendation is not a sound one.

BUT DO WE REALLY *NEED* MEAT?

Beef is often automatically thrown in the junk food category, and many health-conscious folks piously claim they "don't eat red meat" in an effort to avoid heart disease, cancer, and other ailments. The fact is when the pros and cons of any animal product (including meat, poultry, and dairy) are up for discussion, it is essential to differentiate between conventional, factory-produced and traditionally pasture-raised meats.

Conventional CAFO-raised meat is fed improperly, dosed with antibiotics and other medications, and raised in conditions that result in unhealthy, toxic meat. On the other hand, good quality beef—from pasture-raised cattle—is a nutrient-dense, health-promoting food containing no hormones or unnecessary antibiotics. It's a great source of saturated fat and cholesterol your body needs to function properly.

Grass-fed beef and dairy also contain significantly more CLA (conjugated linoleic acid), omega-3 fatty acids, and vitamin E. CLA supports the immune system and may help fight cancer, and both omega-3 fats and CLA in grass-fed beef actually reduce the risk of heart disease. In terms of fertility, omega-3 fats help regulate hormones, increase cervical mucus, and aid in normalizing the menstrual cycle. See page 131 [section on fish oil] for more about the omega-3 fatty acids.

One concern that's valid regardless of where your beef comes from is the temperature at which you cook it. Broiling, grilling, or blackening at high temperatures can cause carcinogens to form on any foods (including veggies), so the best cooking methods are slow, low-temperature stewing or baking, or lightly grilling to medium rare. That doesn't mean you can never barbecue again; just consume meats cooked this way in moderation.

ISN'T ANIMAL PROTEIN DIFFICULT TO DIGEST?

Some vegetarian "experts" claim that humans don't digest meat well, and it essentially rots in the digestive tract. Biology tells us differently: On average, a meal including meat protein, carbohydrates, and fat takes four to five hours to be digested in the stomach. Meat is digested by enzymes produced by our own bodies. Enzymes such as pepsin, trypsin, and chymotrypsin break down meat protein, and bile salts and lipase break down animal fat.

The primary digestive reason we need our gut bacteria is to metabolize the sugars, starches, and fiber—found in grains, beans, and vegetables—that our digestive enzymes can't break down alone.

Therefore, unless your body is not producing essential and normal enzymes and bile salts, digesting meat and fats should actually be much easier than digesting plant foods.

FERTILITY FOOD MYTH #3: EAT WHOLE GRAINS

Many fertility experts make generalized recommendations to eating whole grains to improve overall health and increase odds of conception.

In truth, eating whole grains can be downright detrimental to your health in some cases. Here's why: For women suffering from PCOS and other fertility-related challenges, eliminating wheat can sometimes make a big difference in health and the ability to conceive. But beyond wheat, most grains, beans, and nuts must be properly prepared so that your body can digest them and access the nutrients they contain. If they are not prepared properly (via soaking, sprouting, or souring), problems can ensue.

Whether you're eating brown rice and quinoa or cookies and white pasta, most modern grains (as well as nuts and legumes) are *not* properly prepared. Nearly all of the modern preparations of whole grains that we consume today contain phytic acid that prevents your body from properly absorbing and assimilating the nutrients in your food. Back in the olden days, traditional cultures throughout the world prepared grains with great care by soaking, sprouting, or souring. Our ancestors were unknowingly (or knowingly?) neutralizing the phytic acid in the grains, thereby optimizing their nutritional value. Sadly, these practices have largely fallen to the wayside today.

Improperly prepared grains are likely to contribute to inflammation—exacerbating painful periods, hormone imbalance, and other symptoms of inflammation and pain. Reduce these effects by limiting or only consuming grains, beans, and nuts that have first been soaked, sprouted, or soured. Alternatively, you can eat organic white rice. Commonly thought of as empty calories, white rice can be transformed into a superfood by simply cooking it in homemade bone broth and topping it with coconut oil or grass-fed butter.

FERTILITY FOOD MYTH #4: EAT SOY AND OTHER PLANT-BASED PROTEINS

Soy had a huge heyday as a miracle food in the '90s, and the hype is still alive and well. While soy and soy products might seem like a good source of protein for vegetarians and a great substitute for those who don't consume dairy, in reality, there are quite a number of reasons to avoid it altogether. Eating soy can cause allergies, thyroid problems, hormonal imbalances—including PMS and infertility—and more.

Following are a few specific reasons to avoid soy and soy-based products:

* Soy contains hormone-disrupting phytoestrogens. Soy contains a type of phytoestrogen called flavinones that is particularly destructive to human health. Phytoestrogens are weak plant-based estrogens that mimic the natural estrogen found in our bodies. Flavinones in particular have been linked to early onset of puberty, breast cancer, thyroid conditions, and both male and female infertility.
* Soy contains phytic acid. Like most grains, nuts, and legumes, soy is high in phytic acid, an antinutrient that blocks the body's absorption of essential minerals.
* Soy can cause allergic and toxic reactions. Soy is among the most common food allergens, and it can be a silent villain since allergic reactions are not always immediate.
* Soy is one of the biggest GMO crops. Since the 1990s, genetically modified soy has been widely grown and used in food products in the United States. GM foods pose huge threats on the environment, wreak havoc for farmers' livelihoods, and very likely contribute to infertility.

✳ SHOULD I AVOID SOY COMPLETELY? ✳

Good news for soy lovers: Fermented soy products such as tempeh, unpasteurized soy sauce, miso, and natto are actually quite good for you. The fermentation process neutralizes the phytic acid and flavinones making their beneficial properties available to your body. Fermentation also produces probiotics, the good bacteria that improve digestion, immune function, and nutrient absorption.

That said, you should avoid GMO soy always and eliminate other unfermented soy as much as possible—especially if you are trying to get pregnant, have immune weakness, or have hormone imbalance. Read your labels. Soy is a common ingredient in popular "health" foods and protein supplements. Make sure you know what you're putting in your mouth to avoid accidentally saucing yourself with soy.

FERTILITY FOOD MYTH #5: EAT AN ALKALINE DIET

Many health professionals assert that eating alkaline foods promotes an alkaline environment in your body, which is best for optimal health. Proponents of this diet recommend eating a mostly vegetarian (or even vegan) diet, without sugar and refined carbohydrates. They claim that eating animal products, including meat, dairy, and eggs, will result in an overly acidic body, which may ultimately lead to chronic inflammation, bone density reduction, cancer, and other chronic illness.

While we certainly agree with many of the principles of the acid/alkaline diet, it's not for the reasons you might think. The acid/alkaline diet shares a common thread with the majority of diet plans out there, including ours, to eliminate or dramatically reduce processed food, refined sugar and carbohydrates, alcohol, and caffeine. Beyond that, the acid/alkaline diet misses the mark. . . .

A BRIEF CHEMISTRY LESSON ON PH BALANCE

pH is the measurement of how acidic or alkaline things are, with 0 being totally acidic and 14 being totally alkaline. A pH of 7 is neutral.

The pH of the human body varies depending on the body part it's associated with. For example, your stomach must be very acidic in order to digest food, with pH ranging from 1.35 to 5. Your blood, on the other hand, is slightly alkaline, with a pH of 7.35 to 7.45. The vagina is generally acidic but becomes more alkaline around ovulation, making it more hospitable to sperm.

Our bodies maintain internal pH levels regardless of diet because our survival is entirely dependent on it. In order to keep blood pH steady, the body will metabolize and excrete what it needs to in order to maintain balance. An acidic diet will translate to more acidic urine, but unless you are gravely ill, your vital pH levels (blood and tissue) will not fluctuate by much.

While we give a big thumbs up to eating lots of organic fruits and vegetables and staying sufficiently hydrated, we are leery of any diet that negates the need for animal products of some kind in the human body. Just like the ancient concepts of yin and yang, our omnivore constitutions require that we find balance in our diets, and that they be rich in whole, nutrient-dense foods from across the culinary spectrum. By consuming plenty of fresh fruits and vegetables, mineral-dense bone broths, mineral salts, and fresh water along with properly raised and fed animal products, you are doing more than enough to support long-term acid/alkaline balance in your body.

✳ "WHAT ABOUT EATING *TOO MUCH* PROTEIN? I'VE HEARD IT CAN KILL YOU" ✳!

Many people, including lots of doctors, will tell you that eating too much protein will cause a life-threatening condition called ketosis. This is patently untrue. Health professionals and lay people alike have confused the term ketosis (or nutritional ketosis) with a truly life-threatening condition called *diabetic ketoacidosis*—yet the two things have nothing to do with one another.

Ketosis is a normal body function that refers to the process where the liver takes the fat and protein you consume (and store) and turns it into brain food called ketones. Ketones and glucose (sugar) are the only two things that can feed your brain. Diabetic ketoacidosis, on the other hand, occurs when a type 1 diabetic (or very late-stage, insulin-dependent, type 2 diabetic) doesn't get enough insulin, causing the individual to go into a state of starvation from the inside.

Without insulin, the body can't move sugar from the blood into the cells, which makes the body think it's effectively starving. In an effort to get fuel to the brain, the liver starts making ketones at a rapid rate out of stored fat and proteins. The problem is that because there is no insulin, the liver has no mechanism telling it to stop, and it produces so many ketones that a pH imbalance occurs, leading to serious consequences including coma and death.

Here's the thing: Ketoacidosis isn't actually possible in someone who produces insulin. That's because your body has built-in checks and balances, keeping you in a safe zone known as homeostasis, and in this case, a feedback loop makes sure that ketone levels don't get high enough to change our pH enough to create these problems.

People who consume high-protein, low-carbohydrate diets tend to be in a state called "keto-adaptation." This happens when the body goes from depending on sugar from carbs as its main source of energy to relying on fuel from fats and protein instead. This is especially true for the brain, which switches from glucose dependence to ketone dependence.

In summary, don't be afraid that eating a diet high in well-sourced protein and fat will lead to an imbalance in your pH. A diet rich in these nutrient-dense foods, plus a healthy supply of fruits, veggies, and minerals, is optimal for baby-making and won't do any harm to your inner balance.

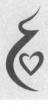

PART 2

Cultivating Fertility

If you're reading this book, we are pretty sure you understand the basics of how babies are made, but when trying to conceive (or for natural birth control), timing sex properly can make all the difference. When we meet with patients we often encounter highly educated, successful women who *aren't quite sure* how their menstrual cycle works, how their eggs grow and develop, or what their best window for conception actually is. This chapter should clarify the confusion about your cycle and conception.

Chapter 1

Understanding Your Cycle

A normal cycle can be broken down into three parts. For the sake of this explanation, we are going to consider a typical menstrual cycle to be 28 days long, even though it may vary by a few days on either side. Day 1 marks the first day of menstrual flow. If your period starts after 5 p.m., day 1 is officially considered the next day.

THE FOLLICULAR PHASE—This is considered day 1 to ovulation. A new follicle is recruited and develops until it reaches maturity. During this time, the uterine lining sheds the old and grows a new one in the hopes of implanting a fertilized embryo down the line.

OVULATION—The brain senses that the egg is ripe and ready to ovulate. At this stage, a surge of luteinizing hormone is sent from the brain to the ovaries, known as the LH surge (a.k.a. the happy face on some ovulation predictor kits).

Typically, the span of time between ovulation and your period takes about 14 days, so in a consistent 28-day cycle, you can usually predict that an egg will be released on approximately day 14 (with an LH surge that happens roughly 36 hours earlier).

It's important to remember that this is only an average. While most women with regular cycles will ovulate 14 days before flow, ovulation can occur 12 to 16 days from when you expect the next menstrual period to start and still be completely normal.

THE LUTEAL PHASE—This is the time following ovulation through either the onset of the period or a positive pregnancy test. This phase is marked by an increase in basal body temperature because the body has to be warmer than usual to host a pregnancy.

In the later part of the luteal phase, you may experience PMS symptoms such as breast tenderness, acne, and mood swings. Pregnancy symptoms are quite similar to those you may experience with PMS, so unfortunately, trying to read your symptoms at this time to determine if you're pregnant is typically futile.

∼ Two Important Tips for Maximizing Baby-Making Potential ∼

Capitalizing on your unique fertile window and making sure your partner's on his game too can go a long way in moving the odds in your favor.

✳ AIMING FOR THE RIGHT WINDOW ✳

If your cycle is irregular or you just want to be sure, you can estimate ovulation using one of the following methods:

OVULATION PREDICTOR KITS (OPKs) test urine for a rise in luteinizing hormone (LH), which precedes ovulation by roughly 36 hours. These kits are available over-the-counter, and while they can be pricey and sometimes unreliable, they are useful tools, nevertheless.

Some kits ask you to start monitoring right at the onset of your period, measuring hormone levels for the full two weeks prior to ovulation. We actually don't recommend these devices. They are expensive and the results can be confusing—frankly, we think they are overkill. By the same token, the supercheap, generic pee sticks can be confusing, too.

We recommend a straightforward, digital urine test stick that lets you know (with a smiley face) when you're in your peak fertility window. When this test is positive, you will likely ovulate within 24 to 36 hours, so time to get busy!

MONITOR CERVICAL FLUID. Just prior to ovulation, cervical fluid takes on the consistency and transparency of raw egg whites. Some women notice this easily when they wipe, while others find the change hard to detect.

For women with PCOS, monitoring cervical fluid may not be a useful method of tracking ovulation, as you may have discharge that is egg white consistency throughout the month, not just at ovulation.

CHECK CERVICAL POSITION. With a little practice, you can check the position of the cervix to determine ovulation by inserting one or two clean fingers. Right before ovulation you will find that the cervix is soft, high, and open—the better to receive sperm. During the rest of your cycle, the cervix is lower and firmer.

TRACK YOUR BASAL BODY TEMPERATURE (BBT) daily, first thing in the morning before getting out of bed. A slight rise (at least 0.4 degrees) indicates that your corpus luteum is kicking in and that ovulation has occurred.

It's important to note that BBT charting is a great way to look at the phases of your cycle *in hindsight*, but not great for in-the-moment ovulation prediction. That's because ovulation has already happened once the temperature spikes.

If you do chart, take them with you when you visit your acupuncturist. Besides predicting ovulation, in Chinese medicine we can use BBT charting for insight into your body's core constitutional patterns.

✳ HAVE SEX WHEN YOU'RE MOST FERTILE

Once you've determined your likely ovulation date, **start** having baby-making sex two days prior to the estimated day. Since an egg typically survives only 12 to 24 hours after being released, the fertility window ends less than a day after ovulation. That said, it is key that the sperm be waiting for the egg when it ovulates, so the true target is the day of your LH surge on a predictor kit, or starting the day your cervical mucus becomes slippery and your cervix moves forward.

After ovulation, many women report a drop in libido and less natural lubrication. Sometimes sex is also uncomfortable at this time. This is your body's way of telling you the baby-making window is now closed.

✳ DON'T FORGET YOUR OTHER HALF

It's kind of a running joke among fertility specialists that if women could take a pill to improve their partners' sperm counts, they would do so happily. For reasons yet unknown to the female species, many (certainly not all) men are resistant to changing diet and lifestyle habits for the sake of their swimmers.

Unfortunately, because sperm issues comprise *at least 30 percent of fertility problems*, resistant men can lead to mighty distressed damsels. So guys, if your wife or girlfriend is forcing you to read this section, please take it to heart. We know you want to have a baby, no one doubts you, but you have to show up for the party. Your better half is going to have to take on the lion's share of this journey, even if the obstacle between you and Junior is a sperm issue. She will still be the one going through the fertility treatments, the ultrasounds, the morning sickness, stretch marks, childbirth . . . need we go on?

Having "unprotected" sex does not ensure a baby. Like an electrical fuse box, there is a trip switch, and while it may seem like you're doing everything right, some couples require a bit of fine-tuning (and sometimes major rewiring) in order for sperm and egg to equal your future child.

✳ SPERM ISSUE? TIME IT RIGHT ✳

If you know or suspect that the future baby daddy has sperm issues, it's best to abstain from sex for two to five days prior to the LH surge and ovulation to allow sperm to regenerate. After that, be sure to have sex on the day of the surge and at least one more time in the following 36 hours.

Chapter 2

Embracing Conscious Conception

WHILE TEENS AND 20-SOMETHINGS SEEM TO GET PREGNANT JUST BY LOOKING AT EACH OTHER, many couples these days wait until they're older to start a family—either by choice (often career-related) or circumstance (like finding the right partner).

It's common for successful women to think of baby-making as another goal to accomplish, but getting pregnant is not like getting straight As or winning a big account. Like it or not, becoming a parent is not something that can be completely controlled.

Plus, the media does us no favors—constantly portraying women in their 40s and 50s pregnant and playing with their babies at the park. What you don't see in the tabloids are the struggles endured, money spent, and avenues taken for these women to become mothers.

We're going to invite you to switch gears just a bit. It's time to make space for a baby. While a bigger house might be nice, what we're really talking about here is making space *in your life*.

Take a moment to consider several simple but profound concepts: happiness, health, harmony in your primary relationships, and a connection to spirit (in whatever form that may take for you). How are you doing in these departments? Got any room for improvement?

Are you a workaholic, barely finding time to sit down or connect with your partner, family, or friends? Do you tend to succeed at most things you set your mind to? Does making a baby seem like another project on your checklist to accomplish?

While getting pregnant requires successful biology, your *humanity* plays a big role in its success. Don't panic—you don't have to become an om-chanting hippy to embrace "Conscious Conception." Perhaps you can carve out a few minutes of quiet time each morning, find forgiveness for a family dispute, or take the time to walk outdoors with your partner once a week. Believe it or not, these actions can calm your nervous system, redirect your health, and improve your chances of getting pregnant and having a healthy baby.

By approaching baby-making from a Conscious Conception perspective, the intention shifts from "achieving" a pregnancy to "receiving" a baby into your body and your life. Not to mention, you'll feel great in the process.

Chapter 3

Self-Care

THE WORLD IN WHICH WE LIVE is profoundly different from the place our grandparents, parents, and even younger versions of ourselves used to call home. The advent of the Internet, smartphones, and 24-hour news cycles have brought the pace of life up to extraordinary speed. Constant bombardment of sensory input means one thing to your fragile brain: stress. While some stress is actually a good thing, too much stress without the time or ability to recover can have detrimental effects on your health.

∼ Managing Stress ∽

The body's stress response is an essential part of human survival—so why is being "stressed out" so detrimental to fertility?

The answer here is simple to state and more challenging to resolve. Stress itself is not the problem. Our ability to recover from stressors quickly and efficiently, however, can make all the difference to your fertility and overall health.

In order to better understand the negative role of stress on fertility, here's a quick lesson in brain anatomy and function: We all have a tiny, almond-shaped part of our primal brain called the amygdala. The job of the amygdala is to make sure we are safe. Whenever stress is encountered, the amygdala fires up, quickly triggering the body to release adrenaline, which starts a cascade of reactions in the body to give a surge of energy and strength—basically calling up superhuman strength to increase likelihood of survival during the emergency situation.

While this fight-or-flight response is exactly what you want while being chased by an angry grizzly bear, it's overkill for most situations. You see, the amygdala operates from an instinctual, animal place. There's no differentiating whether there's *really* an angry grizzly bear or you're just late for work—stress is stress. Issues begin to arise when the body's stress mechanisms are triggered too frequently.

Each time a stressor occurs (such as public speaking, a spat with your spouse, or a car that won't start), our stress load increases. Allostasis is a term that refers to having a low stress load (like homeostasis for the nervous system). If we generally have a low stress load, we should be able to overcome an individual stressor relatively quickly and move on with our day. When we are out of balance or overstressed, each small stressor builds upon the next, until we reach our allostatic-load breaking point. Learning skills to manage and overcome stress *as it arises* is the key to staying in control of your reactions to the challenges life throws your way.

Eliminating stress in our modern world is essentially impossible, but there are measures you can take to manage the stress you have. Give yourself permission to put your own needs first; choose to sit out events that might give you unwanted stress or anxiety; and make self-care a central part of your daily life. Things like gifting yourself an extra hour of sleep, getting a massage, going to acupuncture, and taking time for daily mediation and moderate exercise will all pay dividends in reducing your stress and supporting your fertility.

∼ Meditation ∽

The idea of meditation can be so daunting that many people avoid it altogether, despite assertions that this practice can bring us better health, deeper sleep, improved cognitive function, and improved mental and physical performance.

SIMPLE WAYS TO PRACTICE MEDITATION

Meditation is a term that encompasses many different techniques with the common thread of promoting a sense of inner calm, heightened awareness, and improved health. There are countless types of meditation, from sitting in silence to repeating mantras or listening to recordings of guided imagery. Taking some time to explore these different methods and finding one that feels right to you is your first step toward making meditation a part of your self-care routine. Following are a few easy meditations to get you started.

COUNTING MEDITATION
This simple meditation can help you to slow your mind and calm your inner chatter.

Sit in an upright position with your legs crossed. Put your back against the wall or sit in a chair if it's uncomfortable to sit unsupported, or you can sit on a cushion to elevate your hips above your legs.

Start by closing your eyes and turning your attention to your breath. Begin breathing in and out through your nose. Now, begin to count, allowing one breath for each number, like this: Breathe in and out, while silently saying "one" to yourself, in and out again while saying "two," etc. If you find your mind has wandered to other thoughts or if you lose count, simply begin again from one.

A good goal when starting out is to count from 1 to 25 and back again to zero without letting your mind wander. Increase your count each time you achieve a new goal. Set a timer while doing this so you don't have the distraction of thinking about how long you've been going.

MANTRAS

Mantras are words or groups of words that are considered capable of creating transformation.

"Om" is probably the most well known mantra, said to be the vibration of the universe, which elicits inner peace when repeated alone or in a group setting. Mantras sometimes have spiritual connotations, but they don't have to. You can create a mantra for just about anything. Using a mantra to replace negative thoughts you might be having about your fertility is a great way to train your brain not to stress over things you can't control.

Building on the concepts of a therapeutic method called cognitive behavioral therapy, think about something you frequently tell yourself that might be negative, like "I'll never get pregnant," or "I waited too long to try and have a baby." Next, rewrite that sentence to reflect a positive outcome, for example: "I will become a mother; I trust that it will happen." It may feel a bit hokey at first, but over time, replacing negative thoughts with positive mantras can be very soothing to your nervous system.

TRY A QUICKIE

"Quickies" are our fun little term for mini meditations that you can use to reset your nervous system in a short amount of time and can be done virtually anywhere. Following are a few to try.

MINDFULNESS QUICKIE
Mindfulness refers to the concept of accomplishing a task while paying incredible attention to detail.

For example, try eating a chocolate kiss mindfully. Do this by focusing all of your attention on the task at hand. Start by noticing the foil wrapper. How does it feel to run your fingers over it? Slowly unwrap it, noticing the way the texture of the wrapper changes as you crumple it up. Maybe even roll it into a ball and run it through your fingers.

Next, you might smell the chocolate, or touch the pointy tip. Put it in your mouth and feel it melt or notice how it feels to bite into it. You get the idea . . . 30 seconds of mindful eating is often enough to reduce your allostatic load.

By the way, you can do this with anything, from walking slowly around the block to making a cup of tea or examining a flower. A little focused concentration goes a long way in calming your nervous system.

BREATHWORK QUICKIE

A breathwork quickie will give you a quick reset by clearing your mind through focusing on your breath and reciting this simple meditation:

Go into a quiet room (even a bathroom stall at the office will work). Close your eyes and take a few slow breaths. Next, choose a word for the in-breath and a word for the out-breath. For example, you might choose to breathe in "peace" and breathe out "calm" or breathe in "receive" and breathe out "surrender."

Continue for 30 seconds to a minute. End with a cleansing breath or two.

QI GONG QUICKIE

Qi gong is a martial art that involves gentle movement and hands-on healing. This simple quickie can be done just about anywhere.

Place the palm of your right hand just below your belly button. Place your left hand on the small of your back. Stand up straight, bend your knees slightly, and close your eyes.

Start by taking deep breaths all the way down to the space between your hands. Imagine a small ball of energy floating in the space between your hands, right in the middle of your lower abdomen. See if you can get the ball to subtly move back and forth between your hands. Do this for one to two minutes.

End with a cleansing breath.

∽ Exercise and Mindful Movement ∽
....

Most folks know that exercise plays a key role in keeping stress levels under control. What's more, you can increase the stress-busting punch of revving up your heart by choosing exercises that involve mindfulness or by adding mindful intentions to any exercise you choose.

Yoga is an obvious choice because mindfulness is built right in to almost every style you might practice. Supercharge the stress-relieving aspects of yoga by setting an intention for your practice, such as releasing some harbored frustrations, letting go of fears or anxieties around getting pregnant, or "receiving" a pregnancy (rather than achieving one).

Stay gently focused on your intention as you move through the poses, gently redirecting your thoughts should they stray toward the negative. If you find you can't make it to a class, there are plenty of good videos available online.

Martial arts, particularly tai qi and qi gong, involve following a series of movements, which activate energy channels and can initiate specific types of healing. Find a good instructor in your area or try a video to use these ancient but relevant healing practices to activate the flow of energy throughout your body and release blockages.

Do anything you love. Whether you are walking through the woods or around your city block, sweating in a spin class, or swimming laps, bring in an element of mindfulness and give your nervous system a reset while you partake in whatever exercise you enjoy.

WHEN TO AVOID EXERCISE

Some women worry that exercising too vigorously might dislodge a healthy pregnancy. Generally speaking, if a baby is going to "stick," carrying on with your usual workouts is not going to get in the way.

The only time when a woman should completely refrain from exercise is during an IVF cycle for both the stimulation phase and the two-week wait for a pregnancy test. This is because of potential damage to the ovaries, not a threat to the embryo.

During IVF stimulation, the ovaries swell considerably. The more developing follicles there are, the greater the risk that the ovaries might become very swollen, or hyperstimulated (a condition called ovarian hyperstimulation syndrome, or OHSS). You can read more about OHSS on page 205.

THE IMPORTANCE OF MODERATION

Finally, there is such a thing as too much exercise when it comes to protecting your fertility. In fact, some women actually shut off their body's menstrual cycles from overexertion. From our perspective, exercise boot camps for weight loss are not ideal for women trying to conceive. This is also not the time to train for an Ironman or run a marathon, unless you're very accustomed to doing so already with no effects on your menstrual cycle.

The point here is moderation. Definitely keep moving, but don't overdo it. Exercise so that you feel healthy and balanced. If you feel fatigued, injured, or unwell after working out, it is a sign that you are doing too much. This is not the time to start a brand-new routine of vigorous, high-impact exercise. If you're not at your fitness prime, DO exercise, but choose moderate activities such as walking, gentle swimming, or yoga.

∾ Why Sleep Is So Important ∾

Sleeping is often overlooked as just a means of rest that can be compensated for with a cup of joe, but there's a lot of important biological stuff that goes on while catching your zzz's. According to the National Sleep Foundation, **the average adult woman gets only 6 hours 41 minutes of sleep, when she really needs 7 to 9 hours.** A consistent lack of sleep can have detrimental consequences, both physically and mentally, and may directly impact your ability to conceive.

* Sleep deprivation has a powerful influence on the endocrine system, which can directly disrupt a woman's cycle and ovulation.
* Chronic lack of sleep also leads to low leptin levels, which plays a role in normal ovulation and menstruation, and may contribute to weight gain and a slowed metabolism.
* Sleep deprivation can spike the stress hormones cortisol and adrenocorticotropic hormone (ACTH), both of which can suppress a healthy fertility cycle in both men and women.
* Finally, according to a 2012 study, *Effects of Shiftwork on Sleep and Menstrual Function in Nurses*, irregular sleep patterns disrupt the circadian rhythm, which can also disrupt healthy reproductive function. Women who work night shifts tend to experience more "menstrual irregularities, reproductive disturbances, [and] risk of adverse pregnancy outcome."

MEN NEED MORE SLEEP, TOO

A Danish study published in the *American Journal of Epidemiology* surveyed 953 healthy young men over a two-and-a-half-year period. Men with poor sleep or insufficient sleep had sperm counts an average of 29 percent lower than those men who slept well and enough.

Another study published in the *Journal of the American Medical Association* in 2011 found that sleep restriction leads to low testosterone. After just one week of sleeping five hours a night or less, men had significantly lower testosterone levels (up to 15 percent) than their well-rested peers.

The bottom line: Don't skimp on sleep. Prospective parents should aim for at least eight hours per night, and if you have difficulty sleeping, be sure to tell your acupuncturist so you can work together on getting you some better rest.

∽ Living Your Life ∾

Let's face it—dealing with fertility challenges can be very consuming. You may wake up one day only to find that your life has been completely overrun by your menstrual cycle, timed sex, avoidance of friends and family, and an overall sense of having lost yourself to the hopes of parenthood. If this is you, you are not alone.

Many women complain of losing themselves to the fertility journey, and for good reason. While it's perfectly reasonable that months on end of baby-making efforts can lead to feeling like you have no life, you actually aren't doing yourself any favors by staying on the hamster wheel. We're not suggesting that you should stop trying, but you certainly can scoot your efforts over just a tad to make room for your life that is happening right now.

Consider resuming a hobby, or meeting a friend for lunch and NOT bringing up your struggles, or going on a date or a weekend getaway with your spouse and just enjoying each other's company. All of these ideas and any others you can come up with will actually *help* you in your efforts to conceive, as your nervous system takes things down a notch while you enjoy the things in life that you already have.

The process of cultivating good self-care is not something that magically happens overnight. It's a practice that must be nurtured and tended. While your ultimate goal is having a family, the first step is really learning how to love and care for yourself. Ideally, your future baby should not be filling an empty space in your life, but joining the rich and full life that you're already living.

Chapter 4
....

Building a Strong Support Team

WHILE OUR ANCESTORS MAY HAVE THRIVED IN VILLAGES OR TRIBES, these days we tend to live more isolated, often separated from close family and friends by a long drive or a plane flight. While there may be pros and cons to tribal living, there's no denying that one thing lacking in many modern lives is a sufficient support system.

Because of this common disconnect, we recommend building a strong network of support—via friends, groups, experts, and health practitioners to help to lift and guide you from preconception through parenthood.

∼ Cultivating Emotional Support ∽
....

Women going through fertility challenges often complain of feeling very alone and isolated. Many feel as though they cannot talk about their woes with friends who already have children, or they feel judged and fussed-over by family members. They find little in common with their younger counterparts who aren't yet at the baby-making stage of life.

The longer it takes to become pregnant, especially if miscarriages or other complications come your way, the more likely you are to withdraw from friends, avoiding things such as kids' birthday parties, baby showers, and family functions where young kids are present. While the compulsion to hide out is totally understandable, finding the right kind of support can make the process a lot more bearable.

SUPPORT GROUPS

For many, finding a group of women going through similar challenges can be like finding an oasis in the desert. Suddenly, a world full of people who can truly relate to your experiences become accessible and are usually more than willing to offer you the kind understanding and support you've been missing.

While online chat groups may seem like the easiest place to meet other women experiencing similar fertility struggles, these groups can also be filled with false, misleading, and secondhand information. Regardless of whether you find them to be helpful, we actually discourage spending too much time in these forums unless you can find one moderated by a medical professional.

Resolve is a national organization offering peer-led infertility support groups. The benefit of in-person support groups is the important element of human connection. Many women find great comfort in meeting and connecting with others who are facing challenges similar to their own. Still, like online forums, peer-led support groups where medical advice is dispensed can be confusing and even detrimental, so please be aware of this when participating in these meetings.

The best choice, in our opinion, is a professionally led group facilitated by a therapist or other well-trained health professional. These meetings will often also incorporate the teaching of stress-busting techniques such as mediation and provide an objective perspective that might be missing from peer-led groups.

INDIVIDUAL AND COUPLES THERAPY

Given what we know about the impact that fertility challenges have on women and their partners, it's no wonder there are plenty of therapists who specialize in this important topic.

If you've never been in therapy before, it can feel scary to start, but it's worth overcoming your fear. Fertility issues can take a big toll on relationships, and a good therapist will facilitate keeping the channels of communication open between you and your partner, helping to guide you toward honestly discussing the impact of this process on each of you, both as individuals and as a couple. During this, or any other serious life challenge, seeking the support of a qualified professional is a worthwhile investment of time and money.

~ Calling on Chinese Medicine ~

Practitioners of Chinese medicine learn a vastly different way of viewing the human body and supporting health. This medicine treats the whole person, not just symptoms, and as such can bring a refreshing perspective and effective approaches to fertility. In many cases, Chinese medicine can also find hope and solutions where Western medicine is empty-handed.

For those acupuncturists who wish to be successful in treating infertility, it is essential to acquire a thorough understanding of Western diagnosis and treatments, in addition to the Chinese medicine side, so as to avoid leading patients down the wrong treatment path. When choosing your Chinese medicine practitioner, be sure to ask about their training and experience with infertility.

Training in Chinese medicine is very broad, and most people leave with a degree that enables them to go in just about any direction they choose. This can sometimes pose a problem when it comes to fertility, as this specialty requires a unique skill set, beyond what is taught in a typical Chinese medicine curriculum. Just because an acupuncturist says they treat fertility issues doesn't mean they have the scope of knowledge required to really help someone if things get complicated.

If you are seeing a reproductive endocrinologist, asking him or her for a referral can be a good place to start. Chances are they won't recommend someone who isn't familiar with the ins and outs of their world. Friends who've been through fertility treatments while using acupuncture can also be a good choice. Finally, The American Board of Oriental Reproductive Medicine (www.aborm.org) has a list of board certified fellows who have demonstrated competency in the field of integrative reproductive medicine, through a board exam and ongoing continuing education requirements.

∼ Deciding When to Get Medical Support ∽

While virtually every hopeful parent wishes to achieve pregnancy the old-fashioned way, it's important to know when to seek diagnostic care and possibly medical intervention. Doing so can often save you valuable time and resources in the long run.

Making a baby technically takes two people (or, more specifically, one sperm and one egg). If you are having health issues, are "older," or are encountering challenges, it's a good idea to get support sooner than later.

As a general rule of thumb, a couple is considered to have fertility issues when they are:

* Under 35 and have been trying to conceive for more than a year unsuccessfully
* Over 35 and have been trying to conceive for more than six months unsuccessfully
* Over 40 and have been trying to conceive for more than three months unsuccessfully

While these parameters are reasonable for many individuals, it is also important to consider family history and personal medical history in deciding when to go in for a workup. For example, if your mother and grandmother experienced early menopause and you are in your early thirties, you might consider getting evaluated after three to six months of trying, rather than a year. If you have very irregular periods, struggle with weight management, and/or have to manage hair on your body in typically male areas (such as your chin or chest), you might want to go to the doctor to rule out PCOS (a condition we cover on page 170).

✳ CAN MY GYNECOLOGIST BE MY FERTILITY SPECIALIST? ✳

Sadly, in the United States, most fertility services are not covered through insurance, and many people turn to their regular providers to try to get some of the lab costs and procedures billed. While it is quite common these days that OB-GYNs (obstetrician-gynecologists) offer fertility services such as IUI cycles, it is our experience that this is not always the best route to take.

We often see a number of issues arise when a patient opts for using an OB instead of a reproductive endocrinologist including:

- **INSUFFICIENT MONITORING** through ultrasound can sometimes lead to inseminating on the wrong day.
- **LIMITED AVAILABILITY.** Unlike fertility specialists, OB-GYNs typically don't hold office hours on the weekends, which can leave a woman who is ovulating on a Saturday completely out of luck.
- **OVERUSE OF THE DRUG CLOMID** (Clomiphene Citrate) without sufficient workup to determine if it is the best drug for the patient. Clomid is often used by OB-GYNs as a first line of defense for just about anybody having trouble conceiving, even when they have symptoms that would make its use ill advised (such as low estrogen levels or a thin uterine lining).

On the other hand, board certified reproductive endocrinologists/infertility specialists (RE) spend their days implementing fertility protocols, are generally more focused on finding the right medications for their patients, monitor their patients' progress carefully throughout the cycle, and inseminate at the exact right moment—even if it's a Sunday.

In the world of fertility medicine (at least in the United States), you get what you pay for, and in this case, it's worth the investment. If your case is complicated, or if you've been through more than two or three unsuccessful IUIs under your OB-GYN's care, please consider seeing a specialist.

Chapter 5

Chinese Medicine and Fertility

CHINESE MEDICINE, ALSO COMMONLY CALLED ORIENTAL MEDICINE, IS ONE OF THE WORLD'S MOST ANCIENT HEALING SYSTEMS. It's been used to maintain and restore vibrant health to men, women, and children of all ages for more than 4,000 years.

Today, prominent health organizations such as the U.S. National Institutes of Health (NIH) and the World Health Organization (WHO) recognize the benefits of Chinese medicine and endorse its practice as a safe, valid, and effective form of medicine for many medical conditions.

When it comes to the treatment of infertility, Chinese medicine has a great deal to offer. Before we head into the details of fertility care through this lens, let's cover the basics.

∾ The Basics of Chinese Medicine ∾

The Chinese medical model differs greatly from its Western counterpart. Chinese medicine is a holistic system that uses its tools to promote balance, synergy, and overall health in the body, whereas Western medicine tends to view problems in the body as individual malfunctions that can be individually addressed through medications.

Let's take a look at some of the component theories of Chinese medicine and how they can be applied to the treatment of infertility.

YIN AND YANG

The basic concepts of Chinese medicine correlate to the Taoist view of the universe. According to Taoist philosophy, everything in existence is created through the union of two forces, called Yin and Yang. These forces, or energies, are simultaneously opposite and complementary to each other—much like day and night, male and female, dry and wet, winter and summer, and cold and hot.

When Yin and Yang are in balance and relating appropriately within an individual, harmony exists and good health results. Disharmony or an imbalance between Yin and Yang produces disease and ill health. The aim of Chinese medicine is to restore balance where it is lacking. In Western science, the equivalent concept is homeostasis.

THE THREE TREASURES: QI, JING, AND SHEN

Acupuncture, Chinese herbal treatments, nutrition and lifestyle recommendations, as well as other specialized Chinese medical therapies are used to promote health by supporting and protecting the three treasures: Qi, Jing, and Shen. From these three treasures spring all of the body's physical and mental functions. The way we care for ourselves through lifestyle, nutrition, and mental health plays a vital role in our longevity and our fertility.

QI

According to the Chinese medical model, our bodies contain a series of passageways, much like our circulatory or nervous systems. Not unlike the electrical impulses of our nerves or the blood flow in our vessels, these superhighways, called meridians, are filled with Qi. An excellent metaphor for the function of Qi is to consider that the body is a sailboat; the Qi is the wind that makes it go. Without Qi, the structure of the boat remains, though it is virtually useless without wind in its sails.

The meridian system is the body's energetic circulatory system, whereby Qi, the body's vital energy, travels. Each of the meridians intersects with one or more of the organs, as well as the other major systems throughout the body.

If the flow of Qi throughout these systems is disrupted, blocked, or out of balance, disease, illness, or pain results. Practitioners of Chinese medicine are able to evaluate imbalances in the body by evaluating the state of Qi within the meridians. The restoration of the healthy flow of Qi brings balance that allows the body to naturally heal itself.

The foods we eat are transformed into Qi by the digestive system (the Spleen and Stomach in Chinese medicine terms) and then subsequently into blood and other body fluids necessary for our survival.

JING

At the moment of conception, the energies of the mother and father meet, joining forces to supply their future offspring with all of the resources required to live life. At this moment, a substance called Prenatal Jing is bestowed upon the child, and with it, all the potential for his or her upcoming life.

Prenatal Jing is finite and precious, and once used up, it is gone and cannot be replaced, thereby reducing vitality and quality of life. You might equate Prenatal Jing with your genetic blueprint, which can be impacted by the lifestyle choices you make, how happy you feel, and how healthfully you live (the Western correlation to this is epigenetics).

Jing can be supplemented after you are born through Postnatal Jing—healthy diet, adequate rest, cultivation of a spiritual practice (such as meditation or qi gong), and enjoying a happy life with healthy relationships. Conversely, Jing can be used up before its time, through drug and alcohol abuse, unhealthy diet, excess stress, inadequate rest, and unhealthy relationships. Supporting your Jing through lifestyle is not only important for your own health and longevity—but your future offspring also depend on it.

SHEN

The third treasure in the Chinese medical trifecta is Shen, or spirit.

Chinese medical theory explains that our bodies house five spirits, of which Shen is essentially the team captain. Housed in the Heart, the Shen is responsible for our emotions and our mental health. An imbalance in the Shen, if left unchecked, can give rise to anxiety, depression, or more severe forms of mental illness such as bipolar disorder or schizophrenia.

～ The Five Elements ～

There's an entire school of acupuncture dedicated to explaining Chinese medicine through a lens called the Five Elements. We are going to make it short and sweet here so you get a functional understanding.

Just as the universe is divided into the ebb and flow of Yin and Yang, the Five Elements are another way of viewing and explaining the characteristics and changes of the world around you (the macro) and your body (the micro).

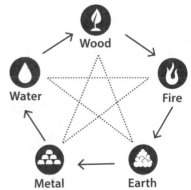

Each of the elements has their own season, flavor, emotion, organ and meridian system, etc. The elements cycle continuously into each other and also control each other like a set of checks and balances.

When one element is off, it directly affects the others—thus explaining the interdependence of all things, including what it is to be human. For example, if the nervous system is taxed from too much stress (Wood), it overacts on the digestive system (Earth) creating upset stomach, poor digestion, gas/bloating, etc.

Below you can see a summary of the characteristics of the Five Elements:

FIRE—Heart/Small Intestine (and Uterus): joy, passion, and spicy

EARTH—Spleen/Stomach: digestion, worry and overwork, and sweet

METAL—Lungs/Large Intestine: immune system, grief, pungent, and elimination (through respiration, sweat, and healthy bowel function)

WATER—Kidneys/Urinary Bladder: adrenals, reproductive capacity, fear, and salty

WOOD—Liver/Gallbladder: nervous system, anger, frustration, and sour

∼ Health through the Chinese Medicine Lens ∼

With a basic understanding of the principles of Chinese medicine, we can look a bit closer at how this medical model is used in treatment, including fertility. Each organ system plays a role in fertility to a greater or lesser degree, and imbalances in these systems also impact Yin, Yang, Qi, Jing, and Shen.

Using acupuncture, herbs, and nutrition, we are able to access and treat imbalances in these systems through their corresponding meridians, called the Primary Channels. While the organ systems come in pairs, you'll notice that we don't always talk about both pairs equally. Instead, we're focused on the organs that relate most to fertility issues.

THE KIDNEY/URINARY BLADDER SYSTEM

The Kidney/Urinary Bladder system nearly always plays a role in reproductive health because this system houses Jing (or Essence)—the deep trust fund of potential energy we inherit at birth. The Kidneys also play a role in creating the uterine lining (along with the heart, spleen, and liver).

Common symptoms of Kidney disharmonies include the following:

KIDNEY YIN DEFICIENCY: When your Kidney Yin wanes, symptoms may appear as lower back or knee pain, ear ringing or dizziness, prematurely graying hair, vaginal dryness, scanty cervical fluid at the time of ovulation, elevated FSH, night sweats, hot flashes, fearful behavior, and a lack of or shiny tongue coating.

KIDNEY YANG DEFICIENCY: Symptoms of low Kidney Yang include sore lower back and knees, frequent diarrhea or loose/urgent morning bowel movements, profuse vaginal discharge, menstrual cramps that feel better when heat is applied, low motivation levels, and a wet, swollen, and pale tongue.

THE SPLEEN/STOMACH SYSTEM

The Spleen/Stomach system encompasses the digestive system, making it essential to assimilating nutrients from food, which bolsters our Kidney Jing and the health of our Blood. This system also relates to metabolic function (including the thyroid) and can lead to anxiety and overthinking if out of balance.

Common symptoms of Spleen disharmonies include the following:

SPLEEN QI DEFICIENCY: Symptoms of a lagging Spleen system include fatigue, cravings for sweets, loose stools, digestive issues, poor circulation, easy bruising, varicose veins, hemorrhoids, polyps, and uterine, rectal, or other organ prolapse.

Menstruation may be thin, watery, or profuse, and fatigue may be worse around ovulation and menstruation, with a possible sensation of bearing-down along with menstrual cramps. Hypothyroid, anemia, and frequent colds and flus or allergies are also signs of Spleen Qi deficiency. Obsessive thinking and excessive worry are hallmark emotions of a weak Spleen.

SPLEEN YANG DEFICIENCY: A Spleen Yang deficiency diagnosis encompasses all of the above symptoms with the addition of cold hands and feet and feeling cold in general. Both Spleen Qi and Spleen Yang deficient tongues are likely to be pale and swollen with teeth marks on the side.

THE LIVER/GALLBLADDER SYSTEM

The Liver/Gallbladder system can be viewed in part as our nervous system, and a happy nervous system is directly linked to good digestive function, healthy gene expression, and optimal fertility. This Liver/Gallbladder system is responsible for the smooth flow of Qi in the body, and deficiency or stagnation in these meridians can results in emotional disharmony, irritability, and anger.

The Liver also has a strong connection to the menstrual cycle, and we say it is responsible for "storing" Blood. A balanced Liver meridian means minimal premenstrual symptoms, because the smooth flow of liver Qi keeps the hormones in check—minimizing things such as breast tenderness, irritability, and emotional upset.

Common symptoms of Liver disharmonies include the following:

LIVER QI STAGNATION: Stagnant Liver Qi shows up as excessive irritability, PMS, anger/rage, pain around ovulation, breast tenderness, nipple pain or discharge, elevated prolactin levels, a bitter taste in the mouth, and/or heartburn.

LIVER BLOOD STAGNATION: This disharmony can present as painful periods, especially when the pain radiates to the external genitalia; dark, thick, clotted, or purplish menstrual blood; and a dark or purplish tongue. It's important to note that Blood stagnation can appear anywhere in the body, not just in the liver system. Hallmarks of general Blood stagnation include pain that is fixed, sharp, and severe.

LIVER BLOOD DEFICIENCY: Light periods, dry skin and hair, a pale complexion, dizziness, floaters in your field of vision, muscle weakness, cramps or spasms, prematurely graying hair, and a pale tongue are all signals that Liver blood may be deficient. Because of the interconnectedness of all things, it's important to note that if the Spleen isn't assimilating enough nutrients, then the Blood will also be deficient.

GALLBLADDER DISHARMONY: The Gallbladder is considered the seat of courage in Chinese medicine. A disharmony in this organ can impact one's ability to make decisions and act on them. The Gallbladder channel also runs the entire length of the body, with much of the channel intersecting with the brain. It is for this reason that the Gallbladder channel can have a direct impact on the hypothalamus and the pituitary.

THE LUNG/LARGE INTESTINE SYSTEM

The Lung/Large Intestine system encompasses the immune system and skin health, and having healthy immune function is essential to successful baby-making. The Lungs also play a special and little-discussed role as the organ of "inspiration." Balance in this meridian will assist a hopeful mother to "call in" the spirit of her baby. Mother Nature is no dummy, and she typically won't give the green light on baby-making to a body that is not processing nutrients, is overrun with stress hormones, or is unable to protect itself from pathogens.

When the Lung and Large Intestine systems are compromised, problems of the immune system occur—including immunologic infertility, allergies, skin issues, and conditions pertaining to the large intestine, such as colitis, IBS, and chronic constipation. The emotion associated with this organ pair is grief and the capacity to let go, often a very difficult roadblock for folks struggling with fertility challenges.

THE HEART/SMALL INTESTINE SYSTEM

The Heart/Small Intestine system (which includes the Pericardium and Triple Warmer, similar to the lymphatic system) houses the Shen, a.k.a. the spirit. The Heart and Shen also have a powerful connection to the uterus and the endocrine system. In fact, it is asserted that Heart Blood flows directly down to the uterus to nourish a developing fetus, forming a profound connection between mother and child long before birth. The Five Element relationship between Fire (Heart) and Water (Kidney) also mirrors the Western correlation between the endocrine system (Heart) and the reproductive system (Kidney).

Heart System Disharmonies: Common symptoms of Heart system imbalance include heart palpitations, anxiety, panic attacks, nightmares, restlessness and agitation, waking early in the morning and being unable to get back to sleep, excessive sweating, especially on the hands, feet, or chest, and a lack of joy for life. The tongue will often have a central crack that extends to the tip, which is likely to be red.

THE EIGHT EXTRAORDINARY MERIDIANS

The organ systems (a.k.a. the Primary Channels) are not the only approach to treating the body through acupuncture. Another system, called the Secondary Vessels, is used by many practitioners worldwide. These vessels have been used since the inception of Chinese medicine and represent a powerful way of viewing and treating the body.

Included in the Secondary Vessels is a group of channels called the Eight Extraordinary Meridians. In our private practices, we use these meridians to treat our patients more than any others because they have a very powerful impact on fertility and emotions and are the only channels that can directly impact fetal health, according to classical Chinese medical texts. These channels impact every level of energy in the body, and we find they are able to bring about healing on a deeper level than Primary Channel treatments.

✳ THE BALANCING ACT ✳

Chinese medicine is like a web or matrix, so changes in any of these systems affect the rest. If you tug on or break a part of a spider's web, the integrity of the entire structure is affected. Likewise, by bringing healing and balance to one area of the body, you begin to positively affect your whole person as well.

Because of the way these channels work in the body, they are able to impact sperm and egg development more directly than the primary channels, with the added benefit of addressing stress levels and emotional imbalances.

∾ The Yin and Yang of Your Monthly Cycle ∾

Whether you are just at the beginning of your journey to becoming a parent or experiencing challenges that require medical intervention, Chinese medicine provides support by addressing the specific disharmonies you are experiencing. Herbal formulas and acupuncture can bring the reproductive system into balance, supported by the lifestyle and dietary changes you will make in your daily life.

The Yin/Yang theory elegantly applies to a woman's monthly cycle, helping to both explain and provide direction for healing.

Below is a basal body temperature (BBT) chart. BBT charts were mentioned briefly on page 31, and whether or not you choose to use them to track your ovulation, it makes a handy visual illustration of the Yin and Yang phases of the menstrual cycle.

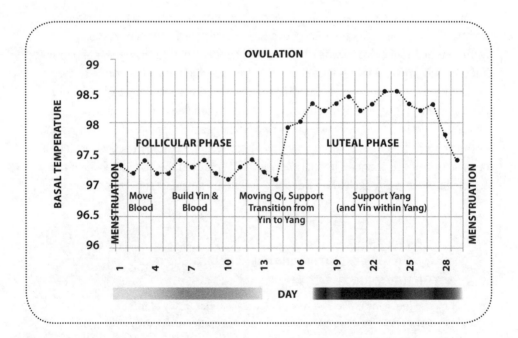

Day 1 is considered the first day of menstrual flow. In a normal month for a menstruating woman, the first half of your cycle is called the follicular phase, while the second half (post ovulation) is called the luteal phase.

Generally speaking, the follicular phase of the cycle is dominated by Yin. This is because Yin is the aspect of ourselves that is *substantial*: our fluid, tissues, and flesh. Because the first half of the cycle is about the thickening of the lining and development of a follicle, Yin dominates. Still, Yang is ever present, just to a lesser degree.

At midcycle, or ovulation time, the Liver is responsible for moving Qi in the ovaries, which allows for ovulation to occur smoothly. The luteal phase of the cycle is dominated by Yang—responsible for both the motive force and the heat within our bodies. This phase starts with ovulation—a Qi and Yang activity—and is maintained by progesterone, a Yang hormone.

At the end of the cycle, if pregnancy has not occurred, the Liver will once again mobilize Qi and Blood to bring on the period. If the liver is in balance, this will occur with little PMS or menstrual pain.

∾ Herbs and Acupuncture for Fertility ∾

Chinese herbs and acupuncture can be used to support the phases of the menstrual cycle, regulating any areas that are out of balance. This system of treating to regulate the menstrual cycle is often referred to as "phasic treatment."

For the sake of simplicity, let's just assume you have a 28-day cycle. In that case, on average:

DAYS 1–5 ARE MENSTRUATION. Your uterine lining is shedding, and the intent with Chinese medicine is to support this process by "moving and building Blood." Out with the old, in with the new.

DAYS 6–12, MENSTRUATION IS OVER, AND THE UTERINE LINING IS REBUILDING. This phase is dominated by Yin. The intention with Chinese medicine treatments at this time is to help your body to build Yin and Blood in the form of your new endometrial lining and developing follicles.

DAYS 12–14 (OR FROM THE LUTEINIZING HORMONE OR LH SURGE PLUS TWO DAYS) IS APPROXIMATELY OVULATION TIME. We support this time by moving Liver Qi and Blood and assisting the body's transformation from Yin to Yang. This transition occurs during and right after ovulation when the corpus luteum starts making progesterone, the hormone that is responsible for higher body temperatures in the luteal phase.

DAYS 15–28 ARE POST OVULATION, WHICH IS ALSO CALLED THE LUTEAL PHASE. Progesterone is high, keeping your temperature elevated. If implantation occurs (usually around day 21), the cells are dividing and multiplying. This phase of the cycle is dominated by

Yang (progesterone), and treatments are often focused on Yang support. **If you have a positive pregnancy test,** Chinese medicine treatments center on continuing support of Yang to "secure the fetus." **If you have a negative pregnancy test,** Chinese medicine treatments aim to move Blood and Qi in preparation for your period.

For women who have regular, healthy cycles, the intent of Chinese medicine treatments should be to simply continue to support the phases of the cycle while addressing any other imbalances or health issues that may be presenting. For women who have irregular cycles or are not ovulating at all, we aim to restore regular ovulation and a normal menstrual cycle.

Specifically, multiple studies show that acupuncture alone or in combination with herbs can:

* Increase blood flow to the uterus to promote implantation
* Improve ovarian function, which may help produce better quality eggs and a larger number of follicles
* Reduce the side effects of drugs used in medical fertility treatments
* Decrease uterine contractions, encourage implantation, and prevent early miscarriage
* Reduce the stress hormones and anxiety, which may contribute to infertility
* Strengthen the immune system and support general health to promote a healthy pregnancy and baby

Herbs and acupuncture work synergistically to direct the body to balance. For those who have experience with acupuncture but not herbs, it is useful to think of them as medicinal resources that support the energetic intentions of the acupuncture you are receiving, further paving the way to optimal health and fertility.

~ Integrating East and West ~

Chinese medicine approaches health care in a fundamentally different way from Western medicine. To understand the difference, consider the job of a mechanic versus the work of a gardener.

Western medicine views health care as if practitioners are mechanics whose job is to fix broken parts. This approach tends to focus on and attempts to cure individual symptoms, as if they are the result of a malfunction in one area or "part" of the body.

For example, stomach conditions are treated by giving medicines (or other medical interventions) for the stomach, just as a mechanic might replace brakes when a car fails to slow down or stop.

While a brake job might be just what your car needs if your brakes don't work, the body is much more complex than an automobile. Unlike cars, the systems and organs

of the body work together, rather than in isolation from each other. The "practitioner as
mechanic" model is simply not enough when applied to human beings. In contrast to
Western medicine, the Chinese medicine practitioner's approach is to tend to the body
much as a gardener would tend to a garden.

Chinese medicine addresses the "root" cause of medical conditions rather than just
attempting to alleviate a symptom, or the "branch." If the leaves on a plant are wilting,
it isn't because they are broken and need to be fixed. It's usually a sign that the entire
plant is suffering some sort of physical distress. Successful gardeners will look to treat
and support the health of the entire plant rather than just focusing on the leaves.
Wilting leaves are like medical symptoms. They point to deeper, root causes for health
problems or diseases that Chinese medicine seeks to treat or alleviate.

Chinese medicine aims to correct patients' imbalances and restore health by
stimulating and promoting self-healing. Western medicine often focuses on the end
result of medical treatments or the final outcome of the course of healing. For example,
in a case of a woman who is not ovulating, a doctor might prescribe Clomid—

a medication to induce the ovaries to release an egg. The patient may or may not become pregnant, but regardless of the outcome, the root cause of the problem has not been solved.

By contrast, Chinese medicine focuses on the beginning of the chain of reactions involved in your fertility challenges, aiming to treat the underlying (root) cause as well as help you meet your desired outcome—a healthy pregnancy and baby.

With regard to fertility treatments, sometimes it is best to call on both the proverbial mechanic and gardener. While addressing the root cause of a condition is always the preferred method for practitioners of Chinese medicine, sometimes a little compromise is ideal. When it comes to fertility treatments, a concurrent root and branch approach is often necessary, especially when time is a factor.

Many people come to Chinese medicine after a long period of trying on their own or in a last-ditch effort to optimize their next IVF cycle. The truth is, it takes time to treat the root, sometimes many months or even longer. Most couples aren't interested in taking that much time off from trying, and even if they are, it isn't always advisable.

We will often suggest a short reprieve from ART treatments (up to three cycles or so) in an effort to balance the body and optimize the reproductive, nervous, and endocrine systems as quickly as possible. This can go a long way in improving outcomes the next time around and sometimes leads to the wonderful surprise of an unassisted conception.

After three months (longer if you are younger and/or interested in giving the root more time), returning to an integrated approach may be your quickest route to Babyland. At this point, Chinese medicine is extremely effective in supporting your body, mind, and spirit through the protocols of Western treatment and in many instances can improve results.

Once you have a bun in the oven, Chinese medicine is also a wonderful tool for supporting pregnancy. It assists with everything from miscarriage prevention to morning sickness, swelling, and back pain. At the end of your pregnancy, acupuncture can even help to gently guide your body into an effective labor pattern.

Chapter 6

Adopting a Traditional Foods Diet

EVERY TIME EITHER OF US SITS DOWN WITH A NEW PATIENT IN OUR OFFICES, we spend nearly an hour getting to know one another. We take the usual health and family history and listen to the story of their fertility journey up to this moment.

Then we talk about food.

REAL food is essential to optimal health, but unfortunately, most of our modern dietary habits focus on marketing and convenience rather than true nourishment. Modern foods are overprocessed in a factory, packaged in colorful cardboard boxes or plastic bottles, shipped across the world, and designed to have an unnaturally long shelf life.

Real food is the food we humans crave and have been thriving on for millennia —home-cooked stews, savory meats, eggs with bright orange yolks, cream, butter, seasonal fruits ripe with juicy sweetness, and veggies so fresh you can taste the earth in which they grew. These foods will spoil if you don't eat them—and this is a *good* thing. Unlike modern foods, real food is teeming with life.

You will read lots of different terms in this book that all refer to real food—nutrient-dense, traditional, organic, local, grass-fed, pasture-raised, biodynamic, and more. Don't be discouraged if you aren't familiar with all of the lingo, don't like to cook, think it's too expensive, or feel like it's all too overwhelming . . . we are here to guide you along the way.

Eating this way is not a new diet fad, it's a lifestyle—one that promotes wellness, leaves you content and deeply nourished, feeds the local economy, and supports the health of our planet. This kind of "holistic" healing can bring harmony to your life in a way that no supplements or medication can, cultivating the best possible environment for a baby to grow.

∾ Won't My Doctor Tell Me What Foods to Eat? ∾
....

Your gynecologist and/or fertility specialists are highly trained doctors, attending years and years of schooling and residencies. As you might imagine with all that training, they have little time or focus to become experts in holistic health or the wisdom of traditional diets. Some make efforts to educate themselves once they are in practice, and seeking out these types of physicians can be extremely helpful.

By the same token, while practitioners of Chinese medicine receive a well-rounded, "holistic" education, surprisingly, nutritional training is not as thorough as you might expect.

Whether you have put your care in the hands of your gynecologist, a reproductive endocrinologist, a practitioner of Chinese medicine, or all of the above, it is very possible that no one on your team has more than a basic grasp of the best nutrition for optimizing your fertility, and, unfortunately, modern nutritionists don't either. Luckily, you have us.

While it is commonly recommended that you start prenatal vitamins at least three months prior to conception, popping a few pills each day is simply not enough. The food you eat in the months leading up to conception is equally, if not more, important to your health and the health of your future offspring than a fistful of supplements whose benefits are questionable, at best.

The right foods can help bring balance and health to your body by eating for true nourishment and optimal fertility. We will not be giving you mainstream advice to eat more veggies and whole grains—though we *will* be teaching you how to eat real, nutrient-dense food that you'll actually enjoy eating.

While you may not have a crystal ball to tell you if, when, or how you will become a parent, you absolutely can choose to nourish your body in ways that will help your overall health, improving your odds to boot.

∾ What a Dentist's Discoveries Have to Do with Your Fertility ∾

Whether for buckteeth, overbites, underbites, or just a bunch of crooked teeth, most adults we know have had braces at some point in their lives. Teeth come in a bit wonky, and parents shell out the thousands to straighten them. Besides the cost and a few years of teenage embarrassment, no biggie, right?

While you may take crooked teeth for granted, it's worth considering why they got that way in the first place. Are humans really designed to have mouths that don't fit our teeth?

One man, Weston A. Price, a dentist from Cleveland who practiced in the 1930s, had a hypothesis. Crooked teeth, he theorized, were actually a skeletal deformity resulting from poor diet. The more generations exposed to a poor diet, the more dental, skeletal, and overall health problems an individual would have—including a decrease in the ability to conceive future generations.

Dr. Price traveled to remote areas of the globe and found various groups of people with wide dental arches, uncrowded straight teeth, and minimal tooth decay. These people, whether in the Swiss Alps or the aboriginal outback, all had two main things in common beyond their good health:

1. They were not exposed to modern foods, which at the time included vegetable oils, white sugar, white flour, and canned goods.
2. They consumed a diet rich in traditionally prepared foods, which included animal fats. (This was true even of the healthy vegetarian peoples who typically consumed eggs and/or dairy).

In his book *Nutrition and Physical Degeneration*, Price documented his research and provided copious photographs of these healthy, traditional people versus their relatives and countrymen who had been exposed to modern diets and thereby displaced from traditional foods. The imagery is striking, and it clearly shows a decline in vitality as the diet becomes modernized.

In his travels, Price found that among the healthy cultures he encountered, couples who were planning to start a family often began preparing six months to one year prior to conception with "sacred" foods to boost fertility. They would go out of their way to consume organ meats, eggs, fat, and seafood.

✳ THE IMPORTANCE OF PREP TIME ✳

In her book, *Beautiful Babies*, Kristen Michaelis explains in more detail about the benefits of Weston A. Price–style nutrition for pregnancy:

A lengthy pre-pregnancy prep time gives [the] body a fair chance to detox and heal as well as to consume the right nutritional resources to grow a thriving, healthy baby.

Tribes who lived in the Andes mountain range would send men down to the sea to collect fish eggs they would bring back to their women. Hearty Gallic fishermen living on Scotland's coast would feed women of childbearing age a dish made of fish heads stuffed with oats and chopped fish liver. Hunter-gatherers in Canada, the Everglades, the Amazon, Australia, and Africa would save the liver, glands, blood, marrow, and adrenal glands of land animals for their wives.

Price noted that the mothers in these particular native cultures tended to conceive with ease and experience healthy pregnancies. Their babies and children enjoyed robust health and possessed good bone structure. However, these benefits almost immediately declined when the mother's diet changed to processed modern foods.

Fast-forward to today: Young couples are not encouraged to consume foods to enhance their fertility, and even "healthy" modern diets are devoid of traditional sacred foods. At best, doctors recommend that women take a prenatal vitamin for three months before trying to conceive, which is advice ignored by many.

THE WESTON A. PRICE FOUNDATION FERTILITY RECOMMENDATIONS

The Weston A. Price Foundation promotes a diet high in good-quality saturated fats from pasture-raised animal sources, wild caught seafood, and other nutrient-dense, properly prepared foods. Here are the recommendations for women who are trying to conceive or are pregnant or nursing:

* **FULL-FAT DAIRY**—4 cups total of whole raw milk (235 ml per cup), cheese (235 g per cup), or yogurt (230 g per cup) plus at least 4 tablespoons (55 g) butter per day
* **EGGS**—At least 2 per day plus extra yolks
* **SEAFOOD**—2 to 4 servings per week plus fermented cod liver oil
* **LIVER**—3 to 4 ounces (85 to 115 g) 1 or 2 times per week plus fermented cod liver oil
* **BONE BROTH**—At least 1 cup (235 ml) per day
* **BEEF OR LAMB**—Daily
* **COCONUT OIL**—At least 2 tablespoons (28 g) daily
* **FERMENTED FOODS, DRINKS, AND CONDIMENTS**—Some each day, preferably each meal
* **FRESH FRUITS AND VEGGIES**—Some each day
* **GRAINS**—Only if properly prepared via soaking, souring, or sprouting

In a perfect world, most women would just jump right on board with this diet, but as you may have noticed, these recommendations are a far stretch from even a *healthy* standard American diet.

For many people, the suggestion of eating liver and copious amounts of butter is enough to make their heads spin. Luckily, Chinese medicine can help us make sense of why a traditional diet is ideal for fertility, and how to make sure your food choices are right for YOU.

Chapter 7

Chinese Medicine and Traditional Diets

AS A MEDICINE ROOTED IN ANCIENT HISTORY, the dietary principles of Chinese medicine don't fall far from Weston Price's observations of historically healthy cultures. The principles of Chinese medicine naturally promote unprocessed, nutrient-dense foods and use food as medicine.

As you've probably learned by now, Chinese medicine is all about finding balance within your own inner ecosystem, and food plays a vital role in this experience. Chinese medicine can fine-tune your diet by helping you to choose foods for your specific needs. For example, both you and I might give up junk food, eat eggs, seafood, soups made with broth, etc., but where I may need foods to calm my nervous system and build Blood, you may need foods to warm your digestion or fortify your Jing.

By directing your energy toward dietary changes that include as many traditional foods as possible plus emphasizing foods to support your Chinese medicine diagnoses, you'll help to bring your body into a state of optimal health, so that normal functions (including baby-making) can occur with more ease.

∼ Using the Nutritional Wisdom of Chinese Medicine to Find Your Balance ∽
....

The principles of Chinese medicine are based on the balance of Yin and Yang energies. As women move through their monthly cycles, there is a flow from Yin to Yang and back again. As you move through your days and life, this same ebb and flow occurs as well. For example, Yang energy rises with you as you awaken in the morning and is at its peak midday when the sun is high in the sky. After noon, Yang wanes as Yin begins to rise, reaching its peak at midnight. When you mimic the rhythms of nature in your own body, you are better able to optimize your health and resources.

Determining your individual excesses and deficiencies offers a custom-made approach to healthy eating, bringing into focus the strengths of both Chinese medicine and a real food lifestyle.

≈ Nutrition and the Organ Systems ≈

As we discussed on page 47, Chinese medicine can be broken down into five paired Organ Systems: Kidney/Urinary Bladder, Spleen/Stomach, Lung/Large Intestine, Heart/Small Intestine, and Liver/Gallbladder. For the purpose of this book, you'll mostly find us mentioning one of the two pairs, the one that pertains more to fertility. That doesn't mean that the other pair is insignificant to your overall health, but it may relate less to reproduction.

Keep in mind that Chinese medicine is metaphoric; so don't necessarily expect that the way organ "systems" are presented here will match the modern, Western understanding of organ function. Chinese medicine evolved long before autopsies and MRIs. Nevertheless, the ancient practitioners managed to accurately understand every bodily function that we know about today, even if the organs they attributed those functions to don't correlate perfectly with the explanations of modern medicine.

In Chinese medicine, each system encompasses much more than the physiological aspects of the organs—including corresponding tastes, colors, emotions, and seasons. By combining these Chinese medicine principles with the wisdom of traditional diets, your specific needs will be addressed, and your body will begin making its way to a balanced state, optimal for fertility and overall well-being.

Let's look at the relationship between each organ system and the foods that support them.

THE SPLEEN/STOMACH SYSTEM

There is a common thread between most holistic medical models that asserts that digestion and proper nutrient assimilation are the most important components in achieving optimal health. Chinese medicine is no different, even placing the Spleen and Stomach system (which in modern medicine would also encompass the digestive functions of the pancreas) right in the center of any flow chart of the organ systems. This concept makes perfect sense to us and illustrates just how vital a role proper nutrition plays in our health.

The Spleen system is represented by the Earth element, reminding us that healthy soil (intestinal microvilli and flora) is required for proper digestion and nutrient assimilation. Too much worrying and excessive overthinking are said to greatly damage the

Spleen. This corresponds directly with our notion of a "nervous stomach." The intestinal tract is filled with more neurotransmitters than the brain itself, further supporting the concept that worrying impacts our digestive processes. Talking through your concerns and utilizing some of the ideas in the previous section on self-care (page 34) can start you on your journey toward a healthy, balanced digestive system.

The flavor that corresponds to the Spleen system is sweet. That's not to say that eating a bunch of candy is your ticket to a healthy digestive system. Our real food interpretation of sweet includes Spleen-friendly foods that are easy to digest—healthy carbohydrates, such as sprouted grains, cooked root veggies, and other high-quality carbohydrates—and an occasional cookie.

As with any of the "flavors," you *can* have too much of a good thing. If you don't do well with grains, they should not be included in your Spleen-friendly diet. The ability to digest complex carbs is different for every person and may require a lot of "soil tending" with probiotic-rich foods before you can assimilate them.

THE KIDNEY/URINARY BLADDER SYSTEM

The Kidneys are represented by the Water element, and the flavor is salty. As previously discussed, the Kidneys house our life's essence, so nourishing this system involves focusing on foods to bolster our Jing resources. Nourishing the Kidney system is vital for maximizing fertility, as it is the root of our reproductive energy in Chinese medicine.

The emotion associated with the Kidney/Urinary Bladder system is fear. People who get stuck in their feelings of fear will ultimately suffer from Kidney deficiency. Similarly, sudden shock or trauma has a tremendous impact on Kidney energy, causing it to scatter. The water aspect of the Kidney system invites us to go with the flow energetically, to allow life to wash over us and to move forward rather than being halted by our fears. Feelings of fear/shock around fertility issues abound for most couples facing difficulties with baby-making.

Foods that support the Kidney system can help to nourish deficiencies and comfort the body to support life's essence and manage excessive feelings of fear. For example, a warm bowl of miso soup will bring comfort and calm, drawing vital resources into a stressed Kidney system.

Foods that encompass all of these aspects (Jing, Water element, and salty flavor) will thoroughly nourish the Kidney system. Oysters are an example of a perfect food to nourish the Kidneys. They are Jing tonics because eating an oyster is eating the whole animal, and they are both salty and watery. It's no wonder they are considered an aphrodisiac. If you don't like oysters, "fear" not . . . there are lots of Jing foods to enjoy, as you'll soon see.

THE LIVER/GALLBLADDER SYSTEM

Imbalances in the Liver system are best correlated to being "stressed out" to varying degrees. In Chinese medicine, the Liver is responsible for the "smooth flow of Qi" as well as the storage and movement of Blood, including the menstrual cycle. Painful periods, PMS symptoms, even endometriosis can be attributed to poorly moving Liver Qi, which we call Liver Qi stagnation.

The Liver system is represented by the Wood element, which (like an unhealthy tree) causes rigidity or inflexibility when it's out of balance. The flavor that corresponds to the Liver is sour, which explains why remedies, such as lemon water flushes, clear out liver toxins and promote optimal function.

Because Wood requires healthy Earth in order to thrive, there is a powerful relationship between the Spleen system and the Liver system. If the Spleen is too weak (depleted soil), then the Liver cannot thrive, leading to conditions such as scanty menstruation, low hormone levels, and PMS.

The Gallbladder, the Liver's pair, deserves a nod here as well. The Gallbladder meridian flows right through the brain, including the hypothalamus and the pituitary. As such, it is powerfully resonant with both the nervous system and the endocrine system.

The Gallbladder channel also relates to the uterus, through its relationship to the hypothalamic-pituitary-ovarian axis. An out-of-balance Gallbladder might lead to things such as muscle pain (including menstrual cramps) and difficulty making decisions (such as whether or not to pursue medical fertility options or if you'd prefer chocolate or salty pretzels to combat PMS symptoms).

THE LUNG/LARGE INTESTINE SYSTEM

The Lung system in Chinese medicine strongly correlates to the immune system. The Lung is responsible for creating a protective layer of energy around the body, called Wei Qi. When functioning optimally, Wei Qi prevents pathogens from entering, preventing illness, and supporting homeostasis. The converse is also true, making the Lung system responsible for bringing good things in—which can be seen both literally and figuratively as "inspiration."

In an esoteric sense, the Lung system is responsible for bringing in the spirit of a baby, and thus must be functioning optimally for pregnancy to occur.

The primary function of the Large Intestine is healthy elimination. Personal experience should inform most people that a poorly functioning Large Intestine leads to feeling quite unwell, from constipation to diarrhea. Both extremes can lead to poor nutrient assimilation, dehydration, and internal toxicity.

In an esoteric sense, the Large Intestine can become imbalanced when one has difficulty letting go—either of past experiences and/or traumas or longstanding belief systems that are not benefiting you.

The Lung/Large Intestine systems are represented by the Metal element, and the flavor is pungent, spicy, or aromatic (such as ginger and cayenne). These flavors help to clear mucus from the body, remove excess gas from the large intestine, and support healthy immune function.

THE HEART/SMALL INTESTINE SYSTEM

The Heart system correlates to the hypothalamus in Western medicine, both of which preside over the body as the governor of the emotions and hormonal function. This relationship to hormones is connected to what we call the Heart and Kidney axis, which is roughly equivalent to the HPO axis (hypothalamus/pituitary/ovarian axis).

When emotions are disturbed, hormonal messages can be impacted. For example, we frequently see delayed ovulation in women under severe stress. As you know by now, hormone imbalance can throw off reproduction, metabolism, and virtually every other bodily function, as well as lead to mild to severe Shen disturbances—including insomnia, anxiety, depression, and mania.

The Heart is represented by the Fire element, and the flavor is bitter. The bitter flavor is not favored by the Western palette and for this reason is highly underutilized. The bitter flavor has a cooling effect on the body, can treat inflammation and excess dampness (such as mucus or cysts), and clears stagnation from the liver. Examples of bitter foods include dandelion greens, bitter lettuces, and citrus peels.

Equal to or more important than bitter foods, people with Shen imbalances related to the Heart must strive to regulate sleep patterns and create a regimen of self-care that promotes inner harmony.

～ A Deeper Look at Food as Medicine ～

Now that we've broken down the primary functions of each organ system in regard to fertility, we are going to look more deeply at how we can correct imbalances through food. Please remember that these are general guidelines, and you don't necessarily need to eat *all* of the recommended foods to experience healing.

FOODS TO TONIFY THE SPLEEN (AND HEAL DIGESTION)

We've already discussed in depth that in Chinese medicine, the Spleen system rules digestion and that healthy digestion plays a central role in overall health, including your fertility. Before we can assimilate *any* nutrients, your gut must be healed from any imbalances such as candida overgrowth or leaky gut syndrome. Nourishing the Spleen with foods for intestinal recovery and health should be the first stop on the road to optimal health through food sources.

There are different degrees to which digestion needs to be healed. Do you have food sensitivities, skin issues, or seasonal allergies? Do you get stomach pain or digestive upset or heartburn when you're stressed? Do you have a slow metabolism in spite of regular exercise? These are just some of the indicators that your intestinal microbes are out of whack and need some attention.

To restore and support healthy digestion, your diet should provide you with beneficial microflora, not be too cold, nor too sweet, and include foods that help to heal digestion along the way. Let's examine these elements one at a time.

GOOD FLORA

On the simplest level, your digestion needs an army of healthy microflora in order to properly digest food. To support this, probiotic foods such as these are essential:

* Yogurt, kefir, and raw milk
* Fermented vegetables such as sauerkraut and kimchi
* Cultured condiments such as ketchup and lacto-fermented mayonnaise
* Fermented beverages such as kombucha and ginger bug sodas

NOT TOO COLD

When it comes to supporting a deficient Spleen, it's important to avoid and/or limit raw and cold foods. This means saying no to a salad for lunch followed by a frozen yogurt or smoothie. Not even one of those things is a great idea if you have any weakness in the digestive department, let alone piling them on top of each other.

If you can't greatly limit raw veggies and cold smoothies, be sure to pair them with warm foods. For example, have a cup of bone broth–based soup with your salad, or enjoy some scrambled eggs alongside your smoothie. Eating cold foods at midday is also a method for mitigating some of the effects, as it is the most Yang time, when digestion is likely working at its peak. Still, if you find yourself feeling bloated, gassy, or uncomfortable after ingesting cold things, it's best to avoid them altogether until your Spleen is in better shape.

NOT TOO SWEET

The Spleen system has an affinity for the sweet flavor. While this is true, a careful balance is in order. Too many sweet things, especially sugary foods, can damage the Spleen. Candida overgrowth is an excellent example. People prone to intestinal flora imbalances will find their situation worsened considerably by consuming sweet foods, including whole grains, fruits, and baked goods or candies. This is due to the fact that *Candida albicans,* a naturally occurring gut bacterium, thrives on sugar, causing it to grow out of balance with other bacteria. Cutting out sugary foods and complex carbohydrates, while replenishing your intestinal flora through cultured foods, will provide an opportunity for the restoration of microbial balance.

HEALING YOUR METABOLISM

If you have a history of restrictive dieting and/or excessive exercising, experience difficulty maintaining a healthy weight, or have symptoms of fatigue, cold limbs, and depression—you may have a damaged metabolism.

Dieting, fasting, and restrictive cleansing can lead your body down a path of metabolic confusion, often erring on the side of caution by holding on to fat stores and metabolizing food slowly. While trying to conceive, it's never a good idea to severely restrict calories, fast, or eliminate macronutrients (fat, carbs, and protein).

Help your brain by sending it the message that there is no famine in sight, and it doesn't have to spend energy stressing about the availability of resources. It might sound silly, but it's crucial to remember that the part of the brain that governs metabolism is primal; it can't reason that skipping meals or restricting calories is for the sake of slimming your waistline and wearing a smaller dress size.

Aside from taking measures to heal your metabolism, the Spleen loves foods that are easy to digest, including the following:

* Soups, stews, and congees
* Cooked vegetables with saturated fats (butter, coconut oil, etc.)
* Root vegetables including potatoes and yams
* Properly prepared grains (soaked, soured, or sprouted)
* Chinese herbal formulas to tonify the Spleen

FOODS TO TONIFY KIDNEY JING

As we've discussed, Jing is the finite and precious material that we inherit from our parents at birth—a divine trust fund, if you will. While you're not meant to squander your trust fund, it inevitably becomes depleted over time from environmental toxicity, stress, drug and alcohol abuse, and even too much sexual activity (yup, you read that right). Jing is housed in the Kidneys, and Jing foods are often salty, watery, and from animal sources.

Jing holds within it all of the potential that exists for our lives. It may be squandered or activated based on the choices we make. The bad news is that the Jing we inherit at birth is irreplaceable. Once it's gone, it's gone. Luckily, you can add what we call post-heaven Jing to your trust fund to make up for and enhance the pre-heaven Jing you lose as time passes. Jing foods have been considered sacred in traditional cultures throughout the world for all recorded time. They include the following:

* Organ meats including liver, heart, and kidney—preferably from pasture-raised animals
* Bone marrow—preferably from pasture-raised animals
* Oysters, clams, mussels, and roe
* Homemade bone broth—from chicken, beef, lamb, or bison
* Eggs—from pasture-raised chicken (second choice—free-range organic)
* Human placenta (your own, after giving birth)
* Deer placenta (available in capsule form, close in structure to human placenta)
* Raw dairy products, particularly milk, cream, and butter
* Royal jelly and bee pollen
* Nuts and seeds, including black sesame, walnuts, and chia seeds
* Chinese herbal formulas to build and protect Jing

YIN FOODS

Yin deficiency is a very common problem among women in their 30s and 40s, generally becoming progressively more pronounced with the privilege of aging. Because Yin is fluid or watery by nature, symptoms of Yin deficiency tend to involve dryness—both internally and externally. This can manifest as dry skin, vaginal dryness, decreased estrogen levels leading to light menstrual flow, and dry or brittle hair—to name a few.

Because everything in the body has both a Yin and Yang component, severely Yin-deficient folks may find themselves showing heat symptoms. This is not because Yin deficiency causes heat, but rather that the relative dominance of Yang energy leads to a kind of internal fake-out, with Yin deficiency as the true culprit underneath. Once the Yin is adequately restored, heat symptoms will resolve or be reduced.

People with Yin deficiency should avoid activities that lead to loss of excess body fluids through sweat, including saunas, hot yoga, and other forms of overexertion.

Foods that nourish Yin include the following:
* Fruit—including melons, apples, mangoes, and pineapple*
* Shellfish and their brine
* Fish
* Eggs
* Pasture-raised organ meats
* Soaked, soured, and sprouted grains, including rice and millet
* Gelatin, from pasture-raised animals
* Kelp and seaweed
* Chinese herbal formulas to tonify Yin
* High-quality sea salt—a moist gray Celtic salt is full of essential minerals, which help the body absorb water (Yin) and maintain healthy balance of body fluids. These healthy salts do not contribute to health issues like powdery, white processed salts do.

*Pineapple contains a nutrient called bromelain, which is purported to aid implantation when consumed for five to seven days after ovulation or following embryo transfer.

YANG FOODS

In opposition to Yin deficiency, Yang deficiency creates common health issues for many women in the prime of their childbearing years. Key symptoms include feeling cold, weight gain, painful period cramps that feel better with a heating pad, sluggish metabolism, and low energy despite sleeping enough.

It is important for folks with Yang deficiency not only to eat warming foods, but to stay warm too. Warm baths, hot water bottles, foot soaks, and generally keeping covered up are all good ideas. This is especially important with anyone diagnosed with a "cold uterus." For this condition, include Yang warming foods throughout the day, and be sure to keep your abdomen covered up and warm—especially around ovulation and menstruation.

Yang foods include the following:
* All the foods for Jing deficiency
* Root vegetables
* Pasture-raised red meat and game
* Pasture-raised organ meats
* Walnuts
* Onions, leeks, and garlic
* Herbs and spices including: ginger, paprika, garlic, cinnamon, clove, and cayenne
* Chinese herbal formulas to tonify Yang

FOODS TO CLEAR EXCESS HEAT AND TOXICITY

You can be hot from excess (think hormonal teenager) or from deficiency (think menopausal woman). Excess heat can wreak havoc on fertility, leading to heavy periods, short menstrual cycles, insomnia, and agitation. Choosing cooling foods can help steer the body back toward a neutral state. Some of these include the following:
* Watermelon and pears
* Cucumbers and jicama
* Dark bitter greens—especially dandelion

If you suffer from excess heat and toxicity, it is also helpful to avoid alcohol, spicy and greasy foods fried in PUFA oils, hot baths, saunas, whirlpools, and heated yoga classes.

EATING TO SOOTHE THE NERVOUS SYSTEM

The smooth flow of Liver Qi is necessary for an optimally functioning nervous system. It is not unusual for the fertility journey to lead to periods of anger, depression, frustration, and even harbored resentment. Help your nervous system along by doing all you can to keep your Liver Qi flowing smoothly:

* Eat small, regular meals, working to keep your blood sugar stable throughout the day.
* Stop what you are doing and eat mindfully, avoiding working or talking on the phone while you eat.
* Eat a balance of macronutrients (fat, carbohydrates, and protein).
* Consider amino acid therapy (explained on page 147) to deal with cravings and emotional imbalance.
* Avoid alcohol and caffeine in excess.
* Get plenty of exercise and enough rest.
* Engage in stress-relieving activities, such as meditation, yoga, and deep breathing.
* Support your Spleen through diet and overcoming worries.

FOODS TO BUILD AND HARMONIZE THE BLOOD

According to Chinese medicine, Blood is made by the Spleen from the food we eat. The health of your gut determines its capacity to assimilate nutrients, which then pass through the small intestine, into the bloodstream. From there, these nutrients make their way to every cell in your body, including the bone marrow, where blood cells are made. The Chinese medical diagnosis of Blood Deficiency is extremely common, especially among women. This is due in part to the fact that women lose blood every month through their menstrual cycle.

Once again, the health of our intestinal bacteria sets the stage for the production of vital components of our bodies, which are deeply impacted by the quality and type of food we consume. You'll see below that many of the foods for building Blood also build Jing. This is because bone marrow, the source of our blood cells, is pure Jing.

Blood-building foods include the following:

* Meat—especially pasture-raised beef, bison, lamb, and wild game
* Homemade bone broth—from pasture-raised chicken, beef, lamb, or bison
* Liver—probably the single most helpful food for building Blood
* Eggs—from pasture-raised chicken (second choice—free-range organic)
* Gelatin from grass-fed cows
* Dark leafy greens—rich in essential minerals
* Chinese herbal formulas to build Blood

The quality of your menstrual cycle provides a pretty good gauge of the health of your Blood, especially in terms of its relationship to fertility. Women with severe menstrual irregularities will likely require additional medical support, including acupuncture, herbs, supplements, and possibly biomedical intervention. Nevertheless, including foods in your diet to support your Blood can only serve to improve upon any treatment you might undergo.

EATING TO RESOLVE BLOOD STAGNATION

Blood stagnation shows up in the body as pain and inflammation. A common example of chronic Blood stagnation is endometriosis, a condition where extra tissue grows and implants on the outside of the uterus causing extremely painful menstrual cramps, digestive issues, and other adverse symptoms caused by inflammation.

Women with Blood stagnation should do the following:

* Avoid processed foods, which make inflammation worse
* Determine if you are allergic to common inflammatory foods (such as wheat and pasteurized dairy)
* Increase consumption of foods that are rich in antioxidants, such as berries, grapes, and wild-caught cold-water fish
* Support the detoxification process of the liver with lemon water and leafy greens daily
* Consume plenty of unrefined salt—which will help your body maintain electrolyte balance and avoid dehydration

✳ FOODS TO WARM THE UTERUS ✳

Women suffering from extremely painful cramps with dark, clotted menstrual blood that is eased by heat applied topically might have a condition known as "cold uterus."

A cold uterus is a primary diagnosis of infertility in Chinese medicine, and it can be curtailed in part with warming foods. For the most part, following the guidelines for Yang deficiency will do the trick.

Warm castor oil packs are a great way to bring penetrating heat to the reproductive organs. Simply warm up some castor oil on an old piece of cloth, apply to your abdomen, and cover with a towel and heating pad for about 20 minutes per day during the follicular phase and when you have menstrual cramps.

Chapter 8

....

Feed Your Fertility: Bringing It All Together

WE'VE TAKEN YOU THROUGH THE BASICS OF CLEAN EATING and Chinese medicine when it comes to optimizing your fertility. Now let's get down to the nitty-gritty—an action plan to protect and optimize your body's ability to get pregnant and have healthy babies.

∼ Ditch the Junk ∼

By removing processed, junky foods from your diet, you will make room for food to nourish your fertility, while protecting your Jing in the process.

By junk, we mean most things that come in a package or don't spoil in a normal amount of time. Junk foods tax the liver and kidneys and generally put additional strain on the body that requires energy to process. When you're trying to conceive, this energy is not worth squandering.

When it comes to trying to get pregnant, these "foods" definitely must go:

* **SOY**—contains phytoestrogens that mimic estrogen and can throw your hormones off balance
* **REDUCED-FAT FOODS**—often contain weird stabilizers to maintain desired consistency or—in the case of low-fat dairy—oxidized cholesterol (the bad kind)
* **INDUSTRIAL OILS**—Despite what anyone tells you, canola oil is not healthy. It falls in the same trash bin as corn, soy, cottonseed, and grape seed oils and should be avoided. These oils contain very unstable polyunsaturated fatty acids or PUFAs.
* **FACTORY-RAISED MEAT**, poultry, eggs, and dairy products
* **CHEMICAL PRESERVATIVES, ADDITIVES, ARTIFICIAL SWEETENERS, AND COLORING**—This should go without saying, but chemicals will put more strain on your already taxed system. Eat real food, read labels, and think before you bite.

This may seem like a big task, and we don't suggest trying to fully incorporate these changes overnight. But, little by little, you can morph your diet from one that is full of empty calories to one that is packed with nutrient-dense goodness. We have found that once you begin to acclimate to a diet of real food, your junk food choices will gradually fall away.

∼ Eat More Fat ∼

We've already discussed the important role that saturated fat and cholesterol play in supporting many of your body's critical functions. Healthy saturated fats help to build Yin and Blood, which translates to having adequate cholesterol for producing hormones, supporting nerve function, and making sure the membranes around all of our cells are working properly.

Saturated fat is essential to fertility because it does the following:

* **PROVIDES FAT-SOLUBLE VITAMINS** (A, D, and K_2)—These are essential for health but are deficient in most modern diets. These vitamins are important to immunity, gene expression, bone production, and many other critical functions for reproduction.
* **STRENGTHENS CELL MEMBRANES**—This includes those of the sperm and eggs.
* **PROTECTS AGAINST TOXINS**—Because saturated fats produce fewer free radicals, they don't cause liver damage or impair the body's detoxification capabilities. When the body is overloaded with toxins, inflammation (endometriosis, PCOS, etc.) abounds.
* **FORTIFIES THE IMMUNE SYSTEM**—Short- and medium-chain saturated fatty acids, particularly the lauric acid found in coconut oil and palm kernel oil, have natural antimicrobial properties that provide protection against undesirable microorganisms in the intestines. This promotes a healthy balance of intestinal bacteria, which you now know is the basis for optimal health, including fertility.

Begin to introduce saturated fats as part of a nutrient-dense, junk-free diet. Include the following foods:

* **RED MEAT,** including beef, lamb, and bison that were raised on pasture
* **PORK** from pigs that are raised outdoors—look for organic and forage-fed. Yes, this includes bacon—but be sure to buy bacon that is nitrate-free. Save bacon fat to use as a healthy fat for cooking.
* **WHOLE EGGS** (not just the whites) from hens that have been raised on pasture—the next best choice would be free-range organic, **not** cage-free eggs.
* **COCONUT OIL AND SUSTAINABLE PALM KERNEL OIL** are great for cooking and baking.

* **BUTTER** from cows that have been raised on pasture (such as the commonly available Kerrygold brand)—this butter will naturally be a deeper yellow color than conventional butter and rich in important fat-soluble vitamins. Coconut butter, milk, and cream are excellent alternatives for those who cannot tolerate dairy products.

HOMEMADE MAYONNAISE

Made with unhealthy soybean oil, canola, or other PUFA-laden vegetable oils, store-bought mayonnaise is the opposite of a health food. Homemade mayo, on the other hand, is packed with fertility-promoting fats and tastes absolutely divine.

Our version is made with eggs from pasture-raised hens, extra-virgin olive oil, and coconut oil. We opt for refined coconut oil for a more neutral taste, and because of the stable quality of this fat, it is not damaged in the refining process.

> 2 eggs, room temperature
> 1 teaspoon Dijon mustard
> 2 tablespoons (28 ml) lemon juice
> ½ teaspoon sea salt
> 1 tablespoon (15 ml) whey, from draining yogurt (optional)
> ¾ cup (168 g) refined coconut oil, melted and cooled
> ¼ cup (60 ml) extra-virgin olive oil

Separate one egg, discarding or saving the white for another use. Add the yolk to a food processor with the other egg (yolk and white), mustard, lemon juice, salt, and whey (if using) and blend for 20 seconds.

Using the drip feature on your food processor (there should be a small hole in the food pusher piece—add oil through there), slowly—drip by drip—add the cooled coconut oil and olive oil as the food processor continues to run.

When completely combined, the consistency will be thinner than conventional mayo, but not runny. It should firm up in the refrigerator. Adjust the seasonings with additional salt and lemon juice, as desired. With whey, mayonnaise will impart additional probiotic benefits and will last several weeks in the fridge.

Yield: About 2 cups (450 g)

RANCH DRESSING

Check out the ingredient list on this popular store-bought brand of ranch dressing: vegetable oil (soybean and/or canola), nonfat buttermilk (milk solids, salt, bacterial culture), water, egg yolks, vinegar, sugar, salt, garlic juice, natural flavors, xanthan gum, phosphoric acid, spices, yeast extract, dried parsley, lemon juice concentrate, silicon dioxide.

By contrast, your homemade version is packed with nutrient dense fats and fat-soluble vitamins from coconut and olive oils, egg yolks, and full-fat yogurt. The yogurt also imparts probiotic benefits. Rather than over-processed herbs, lemon juice, and preservatives, you'll benefit from enzymes and vitamins found in fresh, organic herbs and lemon juice.

We opt to use dried, organic onion and garlic powder to give the recipe a more classic ranch taste, but if you prefer more punch, you can use fresh minced onion and garlic for their added nutritional benefits as well.

Juice from 1 lemon
⅓ cup (20 g) chopped fresh parsley
⅓ cup (21 g) chopped fresh dill
⅓ cup (16 g) chopped fresh chives
1 cup (225 g) Homemade Mayonnaise (See recipe on page 75.)
1½ cups (345 g) full-fat yogurt, strained
1 teaspoon onion powder
1 teaspoon garlic powder
Sea salt and pepper to taste

Juice the lemon and chop up the parsley, dill, and chives. Combine all the ingredients in a quart-sized (946 ml) jar. Shake well to combine. Add sea salt and pepper to your taste.

Yield: 3 cups (720 g)

CREAMY DELIGHT SMOOTHIE

Whether for breakfast, dessert, or an afternoon snack, this smoothie is delightful for your taste buds and is full of great fats to support and protect your fertility.

1 cup (235 ml) full-fat raw milk or coconut milk

2 tablespoons (10 g) cocoa powder

2 egg yolks from pastured hens

1 tablespoon (20 g) raw honey

1 tablespoon (14 g) coconut oil melted and cooled or

  (15 ml) cream from grass-fed cows

Place the milk, cocoa, egg yolks, honey, and coconut oil in a blender. Combine well and enjoy.

Yield: 1 smoothie

✳ HEALTH BY CHOCOLATE? ✳

Did you know that chocolate, considered a sweet indulgence by most, is actually a superfood? Researchers from the Harvard School of Public health concluded that small amounts of good quality chocolate may have some pretty sweet health benefits, including the following:

- Significant reduction in the risk of heart attack
- Decreased blood pressure
- Increased insulin sensitivity
- Improved arterial blood flow (think ovaries and uterus!)
- Reduced inflammation
- Regulation of mood and sleep

The flavonols in dark chocolate have been lauded for their ability to slow down platelet clumping in a manner similar to baby aspirin (though milder). So enjoy a little dark chocolate (the darker the better!) as a part of your baby-making diet.

MEXICAN CARNITAS

This traditional Mexican dish is often made in modern times in a massive vat of over-processed, hydrogenated lard or vegetable oil, which are both horrible for your health. Conversely, carnitas made the old-fashioned way with forage-fed pork and lard is a nourishing food and one of the richest sources of dietary vitamin D.

Perfect carnitas are moist in the center and slightly crispy on the outside. Many restaurants achieve this with a deep-fryer. Made at home, the trick is to cook at a very low temperature—no more than 285°F (141°C)—until the muscle meat is broken down so it practically melts in your mouth. To achieve the crispy outside, finish the meat by quickly pan-frying on high heat.

> **4 to 5 pounds (1.8 to 2.3 kg) pork shoulder or butt**
> **2 limes, divided**
> **Sea salt**
> **1 bunch of cilantro, minced and divided**
> **2 bay leaves**
> **3 cloves of garlic, halved**
> **3 whole cloves**
> **2 or 3 small oranges**
> **2 to 3 quarts (1.9 to 2.8 L) rendered pork fat (lard), depending on the size of your pork shoulder and Dutch oven. (You want the pork completely covered). You will need about 6 pounds (2.7 kg) of fat to yield 2 quarts (1.9 L) of lard for this recipe.**

Season the pork shoulder with the juice of one lime, a generous sprinkling of sea salt, half the cilantro, bay leaves, garlic, and whole cloves. Cover and refrigerate for up to 24 hours.

Remove the pork from the fridge; drain and pat dry. Allow it to come to room temperature. Preheat the oven to 285°F (141°C).

Place the pork shoulder in a small Dutch oven (the smallest you have to fit the meat, but with room to still cover it with liquid). Cut the oranges into eighths, leaving the rinds on. Place your orange slices around the sides of the pork.

Warm your rendered lard (if previously chilled to solid) until it is liquid. Pour the liquid lard over the pork and oranges until the meat is completely covered.

Place the meat in the preheated oven with the lid on. Consider setting your Dutch oven on a lipped tray to catch any overflow of fat. Cook for 4 to 6 hours or until the meat pulls apart easily with a fork.

Remove from the oven and carefully lift the meat out onto a dish, taking care not to burn yourself with the hot fat. Pull the meat apart into medium-size chunks and then fry in a large frying pan with the cooked oranges until the desired crispiness is reached.

Serve with a squeeze of lime, a pinch of cilantro, and sprinkle of sea salt to taste. The fried oranges can be eaten, rind and all.

Strain the lard and save it in the fridge (for a few weeks) or freezer (for much longer) for your next few batch of carnitas. The flavor of the seasoning stays in the fat, so each batch gets progressively more delicious!

Yield: 4 to 6 servings

✳ HOW TO RENDER LARD ✳

Rendering lard is actually quite easy. The hardest part may be sourcing a local farmer or butcher who can guarantee your purchase comes from humanely raised pork. This means animals that have been forage-fed and spent time out-doors in sunshine (essential for the vitamin D). Pigs are omnivores, so they will eat just about anything. Their diets should not consist of GMO feed.

If you plan to use the lard for baking, you will want "leaf lard," which is made from the pig's belly fat. You can render your lard from back or other fat for any other cooking applications.

You will need about 3 pounds (1.4 kg) of fat to yield 1 quart (946 ml) of lard.

Cut the fat into 1- to 2-inch (2.5 to 5 cm) chunks. In small batches, pulse in a food processor until ground, or you can ask your butcher or farmer to grind the fat before you buy it.

Place ground fat into a large saucepan, add about ½ cup (120 ml) of water per pound, and cook on high with no lid until you are left with a pan of liquid fat and some grizzly bits of protein. This usually takes 30 to 45 minutes.

Strain the fat into wide-mouth jars until ready to use. (If the jars are narrow at the top, it will be difficult to get hardened lard out later.)

You can also drain and save your bacon grease to use as rendered lard. Just don't use this fat for baking unless you want a bacon-flavored pie. Lard will last several weeks in the fridge and can also be frozen for future use.

You can use your lard in our delicious Mexican Carnitas recipe. Other ways to include this wonderful fat are endless—for sautéing or frying just about anything or as oil for making homemade popcorn. Feel free to eat generous amounts—traditional lard supports healthy hormone function.

SLOW COOKER BEEF AND MUSHROOM STEW

Delicious, easy comfort food doesn't get much better than this. You could take the time to brown the meat and sauté the mushrooms and onions, but this dish is just as flavorful and is much less fuss when you just throw it all in the slow cooker and come back later.

A smattering of barley gives just enough starch to slightly thicken the liquid in this dish. We prefer using pearled barley as opposed to the whole-grain/hulled versions. Though slightly less nutritious, when the bran is removed, the barley does NOT have to be soaked to improve its digestibility. Because the rest of the dish is so nutrient-dense, we don't think twice about this shortcut.

If you prefer a whole-grain barley, we suggest first soaking it overnight and then rinsing it well before cooking.

If you will be gone all day, make sure you have a slow cooker that will switch to warm after the cooking time is done.

2 pounds (900 g) stew meat
1 large onion
2 large carrots
2 pounds (900 g) mushrooms
1 can (28 ounces, or 785 ml) whole stewed tomatoes
A few sprigs of thyme
4 cloves of garlic
2 cups (475 ml) beef bone broth
⅓ cup (67 g) pearled barley
Good quality salt and pepper to taste

Cube the stew meat. Peel and chop the onions and carrots into large chunks. Slice the mushrooms. Drain the stewed tomatoes. Tie up the thyme with twine.

Place the meat, onions, carrots, mushrooms, tomatoes, thyme, garlic, broth, and salt and pepper in the slow cooker. Set to low and cover.

Cook on low for 6 to 8 hours or until meat pulls apart easily with a fork.

After 4 hours, add the pearled barley and continue cooking. (If you will be away all day, simply add the barley when you add the other ingredients.)

Adjust the seasonings with salt and pepper to taste before serving.

Yield: 4 to 6 servings

∾ Give Dairy a Chance ∾

While milk is often demonized as a culprit for many health issues, historical evidence as well as budding research on the benefits of raw (unpasteurized), full-fat milk is encouraging.

In a well-publicized study conducted by the Harvard School of Public Health, researchers concluded that milk is *not* in and of itself responsible for infertility. Rather, "high intake of low-fat dairy foods may increase the risk of infertility whereas intake of high-fat dairy foods may decrease this risk."

In Chinese medicine, dairy is often negatively associated with creating pathological dampness. This may be in part due to the fact that historically dairy was not a common food in ancient China; these people did not possess adequate lactase to digest the lactose, leading to digestive problems. In modern times, the problem of lactose intolerance has become much more widespread with the prevalence of pasteurized dairy products. When milk undergoes pasteurization, essential enzymes are destroyed that would have otherwise helped the body to digest the lactose.

Raw milk from grass-fed cows, on the other hand, is a traditional food that has been consumed by humans for more than 10,000 years. It offers many health benefits, as it is a complete food and a natural source of all the essential nutrients your body needs to function properly.

In its optimal form, milk contains protein, the eight essential amino acids, healthy fats including conjugated linoleic acid (CLA), minerals, vitamins A, D, and most Bs, enzymes, and cholesterol. Raw dairy is even richer in nutrients and beneficial bacteria when consumed in the form of fermented or soured dairy products such as yogurt, kefir, and raw cheeses.

If you've shunned dairy as an unhealthy food, we recommend that you give it a second consideration, as the nutritional benefits to fertility can be profound. Always seek out dairy that comes from healthy grass-fed animals, and minimally processed is best. For information on sourcing raw milk, visit RealMilk.com.

COUNTERTOP YOGURT

With a mesophilic or room-temperature starter culture, you don't need to figure out how to keep your milk warm while it's culturing. You simply let it sit on the countertop in a warm kitchen until the yogurt has set. The consistency still isn't as thick as store-bought yogurt, but it's super easy to hang and thicken the yogurt if you're in the mood for Greek style or even yogurt cream cheese.

This recipe calls for raw milk, but you can also use a combination of cream and milk for a richer consistency, or substitute pasteurized milk (from grass-fed cows) if you don't have access to raw dairy. Viili and other mesophilic starter cultures are fairly easy to find online.

> **5 to 6 cups (1.2 to 1.4 L) raw milk**
> **1 packet viili or another mesophilic starter culture**

Place 1 to 2 cups (235 to 475 ml) of milk in a small nonreactive saucepan over medium-high heat, just until the milk begins to rise up the side of the pan. Remove the pan from the heat and allow to cool. This pasteurizes the milk for the starter so that the beneficial bacteria in the raw milk don't overtake the yogurt cultures.

When the milk has cooled to room temperature, simply stir in your starter culture and allow to sit on the countertop for about 12 hours until the yogurt is set it, and then refrigerate.

You can then use this "mother" culture to make this week's yogurt and to make a new starter culture every week or so. If you keep up with maintaining your culture, you can make yogurt infinitely from this original starter—never having to buy anything but milk.

Once you've made your starter culture, you're ready to make the easiest home-made yogurt.

Take 1 tablespoon (15 g) of starter culture and place it in a clean quart-size glass jar. Fill the jar with raw milk, leaving about 1 inch (2.5 cm) of headspace. Give it a stir, loosely cover it with a small bit of clean, dry cloth, and secure it with a rubber band.

Allow this to sit on the countertop overnight (about 12 hours). In the morning, if you tip the jar you should notice that the milk has thickened into yogurt. If this has not happened, your kitchen may be too cool, so let it sit until it thickens—this may take up to 24 hours.

Transfer your yogurt to the fridge to cool and set, and you're done!

Yield: 1 cup (230 g) starter culture and 1 quart (920 g) yogurt

SIMPLE HOMEMADE CHEESE

Fromage blanc, also known as queso fresco, is a simple and delicious homemade cheese that is essentially just like common goat cheese (chevre), but made from cow's milk. This recipe will work for pasteurized milk, too, but avoid all ultrapasteurized dairy if possible. Mesophilic starter cultures and rennet are fairly easy to find online. You will also need a digital thermometer to monitor the temperature of the milk.

> **1 gallon (3.8 L) raw cow's milk**
> **1 pinch mesophilic culture for cheese making**
> **3 drops of liquid rennet**
> **¼ cup (60 ml) filtered water**
> **Unrefined sea salt to taste**

Pour the cow's milk into a nonaluminum pot and warm to 72°F (22°C).

Remove from the heat and add the cheese culture. Mix for about 20 strokes, taking care not to scrape the bottom of the pot.

Place 3 drops rennet into ¼ cup (60 ml) filtered water. Add to the warmed milk.

Cover and allow to sit for 12 hours at room temperature. After 12 hours, check for a "clean break" (the cheese should move in a solid mass and jiggle like jelly).

Line a large bowl with a clean flour sack towel. Gently pour the contents of the pot (now curds and whey) into the towel-lined bowl. Gather the corners of the towel and wrap two rubber bands around the gathered ends to make a bundle. Hang the dripping cheesecloth over the large bowl from a kitchen cabinet or similar setup.

Allow to drain for 6 to 24 hours depending on your desired consistency. We prefer 10 to 12 hours for a moist but crumbly cheese. Add sea salt to taste.

The liquid that remains in the bowl is whey. It can be stored in the fridge for months and added to recipes to help them ferment, such as our Homemade Mayonnaise (page 75) and Cultured Ketchup (page 87).

Yield: 1 pound (455 g)

SUPERPOWERED CHOCOLATE PUDDING

Who's to say that chocolate pudding is only a special treat for kids? Made from raw milk, eggs, and gelatin and sweetened with raw honey, this fun dessert is a fertility powerhouse.

2 cups (475 ml) raw milk, divided
5 tablespoons (25 g) cocoa powder or raw cacao
2 tablespoons (10 g) gelatin powder
3 tablespoons (60 g) raw honey
2 teaspoons vanilla extract
2 egg yolks

Heat 1 cup (235 ml) milk in a small saucepan over medium heat.

Add the cocoa powder and whisk until the chocolate is melted.

Remove from heat and sprinkle in the gelatin powder and honey and whisk until both the gelatin and honey are dissolved. Beat the egg yolks separately. Whisk in the remaining 1 cup (235 ml) milk, vanilla extract, and egg yolks.

Let the mixture cool in the fridge. When gelled, you can eat it immediately or beat the mixture with an immersion blender or handheld blender to create a smooth, creamy consistency.

Yield: Four 6-ounce (170 g) servings

∾ Incorporate Cultured Foods ∾

Cultured (a.k.a. fermented) foods are deliberately allowed to sour or ferment naturally at room temperature or slightly warmer. Historically, culturing foods was a way to preserve them without refrigeration. Milk was cultured into yogurt and aged into cheese. Cabbage was fermented into sauerkraut and cucumbers became pickles. Salmon was aged with lemon and salt to become lox.

Beyond the benefit of a naturally long shelf life, cultured foods are rich in probiotics. Probiotics are the beneficial bacteria necessary for good digestive health and immune function, which is why they are so important in your fertility-enhancing diet. While our ancestors were probably unaware of the presence of these friendly microorganisms, most cultures consumed these foods regularly. Meanwhile, our modern diet is mostly replete of probiotics (with the exception of yogurt and maybe kefir), and many of these foods (pickles especially) are produced with shortcuts and preservation methods that allow for longer shelf life, but lack probiotic content.

From a Chinese medicine perspective, cultured foods are ideal for supporting the Spleen system, which in turn produces healthy Blood, the foundation of a healthy immune system and overall health.

Luckily, the traditional food and slow food movements have revived some of the practices that bring probiotics back into our diets via delicious cultured foods. At health food stores, it's not uncommon to find traditionally fermented sauerkraut and pickles (such as Bubbies brand), kombucha, several brands of traditionally fermented kimchi, and of course, an entire shelf of yogurt and kefir.

You can find numerous recipes for cultured foods online, and Sandor Katz's book *Wild Fermentation* is a great resource, too. Have fun exploring the world of cultured foods—it's an affordable and delicious adventure that will benefit your entire body.

TRADITIONAL SAUERKRAUT

Sauerkraut is the perfect starter fermented veggie. It's easy to make, delicious, and rich in probiotics. As part of your fertility diet, include at least a few tablespoons (45 to 55 g) of cultured veggies with one to three meals per day.

You can use the following technique to ferment any combination of veggies you like.

1 head cabbage, preferably organic
1 tablespoon (15 g) unrefined sea salt

Remove one core from the head of cabbage. Shred the cabbage into thin ribbons with a knife or food processor. Place the shredded cabbage in a large bowl.

Sprinkle 1 tablespoon (15 g) sea salt over the cabbage.

Knead/squeeze the shredded cabbage for 1 to 3 minutes. Get into it! You are breaking the cabbage down and helping it to release its juices. Flatten the kraut into the bottom of your bowl and lay a clean tea towel over the bowl. Now, walk away and go about your day.

Later (6 to 8 hours or at your convenience), knead your shredded cabbage for 1 more minute, mixing it all together.

Add this soupy cabbage mixture to a fermentation crock or mason jar and press the cabbage down firmly. Really pack it in there. It should be at least 1 inch (2.5 cm) from the lid of your jar and should be covered at the top with the beautiful brine you have made. Note: If you used a large head of cabbage, you may be able to fill an additional small jar as well.

Screw the lid on tight. Plastic lids will allow for expansion with greater ease than metal lids. Place your jar of culturing cabbage on a plate (to catch any brine that may be pushed out) and leave at room temperature (70°F to 85°F, or 21°C to 29°C) for about 4 weeks for optimal probiotic content. When your kraut reaches desired fermentation (tart and crunchy), wipe up your jar and put it in the refrigerator.

Yield: Approximately 3 to 4 quarts (1.7 to 2.3 kg)

CULTURED KETCHUP

It's a beautiful thing when ketchup can be a health food. This recipe makes a quart-sized (946 ml) jar plus about another 6 ounces (170ml), so you can use the extras right away while you wait for the quart to ferment.

Look for tomato paste in glass jars (to reduce BPA exposure). Grade B maple syrup is richer in minerals than grade A. If you can, get Red Boat Fish Sauce (available online)—it is the most delicious one on the planet. If you opt to skip the whey, the ketchup will still be delicious but will no longer provide probiotic benefits.

> **2 or 3 cloves of garlic**
> **28 ounces (785 g) tomato paste**
> **¼ cup (60 ml) fresh whey**
> **½ cup (160 g) grade B maple syrup**
> **½ cup (120 ml) fermented fish sauce**
> **2 tablespoons (28 ml) unpasteurized apple cider vinegar**
> **1 teaspoon allspice**
> **½ teaspoon ground clove**
> **Sprinkle of cayenne pepper**

Peel and mash the garlic cloves. Mix all the ingredients in a large bowl until well blended. Transfer to a quart-sized (946 ml) glass mason jar with a wide mouth for easy access later. The top of the ketchup should be about 1 inch (2.5 cm) below the rim of the jar.

If you used whey, leave at room temperature overnight and then transfer to the fridge and enjoy.

Yield: 1 quart (960 g)

KOMBUCHA

Kombucha is a delicious probiotic-rich drink that's thrifty, fun, and easy to make. Rumored to have originated in China around 200 BCE, societies throughout the world have been brewing kombucha for centuries. It is made by placing a strange mushroom-like life form called a scoby into a gallon of sweetened tea.

SCOBY is actually an acronym for Symbiotic Culture of Bacteria and Yeast, and the kombucha gets its unique flavor and probiotic power because the scoby "eats" the sugar and components of the tea, leaving delicious, nutritious kombucha behind.

A great alternative to juice or sodas, most folks are quick to acquire a taste for kombucha when they don't have the alternative of sugary, junky drinks. If you have a friend who brews her own kombucha, ask her for a scoby baby in about 1 cup (235 ml) of kombucha. Otherwise, you can buy a scoby online.

> **5 to 10 organic black tea bags**
> **1 cup (200 g) organic white sugar**
> **1 gallon (3.8 L) filtered water**
> **1 kombucha scoby**
> **1 cup (235 ml) reserved kombucha from a previous batch (or liquid that came with your scoby)**

Make your tea in the ratio of 1 cup (200 g) organic white sugar for each gallon of black tea. You may need to adjust the amount of tea depending on the brand or variety you choose. If you want to decrease the caffeine in your kombucha, first "shock" the tea bags by pouring hot water over them, allowing them to seep for a few seconds, and then discarding that first tea.

Add boiling filtered water to fill your gallon jar halfway. Allow the tea to steep for at least 5 to 10 minutes until brewed darkly. Add cool filtered water so that your container is about 85 percent full.

When the sweetened tea is cooled to body temperature, add the scoby. Don't forget to add the accompanying komucha.

Cover with a tea towel and secure with a large rubber band. Mark your jar with today's date. Store your brewing kombucha in a warm, dark place away from other fermenting foods or potential mold. Starting around 14 days, begin tasting your kombucha. It should be tart and zingy, slightly sweet, but not cloying. In the winter, you may need to brew your kombucha for much longer than 2 weeks. Try placing it near your (working) slow cooker or near a warm appliance.

When your kombucha is ready, with clean hands, remove the scoby gently from the newly brewed kombucha and place in a separate bowl. Reserve approximately 1 cup (235 ml) kombucha per gallon and add it to the scoby in its bowl.

Your next task is pouring the kombucha into bottles for storage. You may want to transfer your liquid goodness into a spouted bowl to make the pouring easier. Find a good combination of spouts and funnels to pour the kombucha as neatly as possible.

Store your kombucha in glass bottles with tight-fitting lids. For extra fizz, allow the sealed bottles to sit at room temperature for 24 hours before refrigerating. When your bottles are filled, it's time to begin the process again so you will never be without your booch.

Yield: 1 gallon (3.8 L)

～ Eat Properly Prepared Grains, Legumes, and Nuts ～

Nearly all of the modern preparations of grains that we consume today (whole or refined) contain phytic acid and other antinutrients that prevent your body from properly absorbing and assimilating the nutrients in your food.

Back in the olden days, traditional cultures throughout the world prepared grains with great care by soaking, sprouting, or souring. Our ancestors were unknowingly neutralizing the phytic acid in the grains, thereby optimizing their nutritional value.

Some women find that omitting grains (or at least wheat) altogether is best for their fertility and overall health. We recommend that if you're going to eat grains, you only eat grains, beans, and nuts that have first been soaked, sprouted, or soured. The exception to this rule is white rice. Since all of the bran has been removed from white rice, it can provide a benign (albeit simplistic) nutritional source of carbohydrates.

HOW TO SOAK GRAINS AND BEANS

Soaking grains and beans before cooking releases phytase, which allows the phytic acid to be neutralized. Soaking can also make grains easier to digest, as the process neutralizes enzyme inhibitors that prevent the grain (seed) from germinating under poor growing conditions. When soaked, grains are prepared for growth into a new plant. During this process, beneficial enzymes are produced and vitamin content is boosted.

Soak the grains for 12 to 24 hours in water with 1 to 2 tablespoons (15 to 28 ml) of whey, vinegar, lemon juice, yogurt, buttermilk, or kefir. Rinse well to remove any acidic taste and cook as usual in fresh water.

Soaking grains is the easiest way to reduce their phytic acid—it just takes a bit of discipline. Every night after dinner or before bed, scoop your grains in a bowl and top with filtered water. In the morning, you will have oats, rice, or grain of your choosing ready to go.

HOW TO SPROUT GRAINS AND BEANS

Sprouting grains transforms them into food of superior nutritious value. In addition to neutralizing phytic acid, sprouting activates food enzymes and increases vitamin content. Sprouted grain has more protein and less starch compared to nonsprouted grain, and it has a lower glycemic index value.

To sprout grains, choose high-quality, organic grains and rinse them thoroughly. Place in a ceramic pot or glass jar and add enough filtered warm water to cover all grains by several inches. Soak the grains overnight; then drain and rinse well. Rinse them several times the first day and continue rinsing them until they have sprouted. Rinse and drain before using, refrigerating, or dehydrating to make sprouted flour.

While homemade is usually best because you know where your grains came from and how they were prepared, most well-stocked health food stores sell delicious sprouted breads and crackers. You can find wonderful sprouted flour for baking, including gluten-free options such as sprouted rice, quinoa, and buckwheat flours.

SOURING GRAINS

The most classic example of soured grain is sourdough bread, which is delicious and digestible food if you are eating wheat, but it can also be made with gluten-free ingredients if you are feeling ambitious. Souring neutralizes phytic acid. Souring or lactic acid fermentation enhances the body's ability to take advantage of the nutrients in grains (as well as other foods).

Typically, grains are soaked and allowed to sour for between 12 hours and several days. Most sourdough bread found in restaurants and grocery stores is not prepared with traditional souring time, and therefore does not have the same health benefits. Read the label: It should NOT list yeast as one of the ingredients, which is an indicator that the bread was not made with a proper sourdough starter. In the United States,

Whole Foods Market carries several traditional (wheat) sourdough options, so if you're eating wheat, this is an easy place to start.

HOW TO PROPERLY PREPARE NUTS

Nuts contain plenty of good nutrition, but they also contain antinutrition in the forms of phytic acid AND enzyme inhibitors, which make the nuts difficult to digest and block the absorption of minerals. Phytic acid and enzyme inhibitors can be neutralized by first soaking and then drying nuts before eating them or using them to make butters or flours. Unfortunately, even organic nut butters—regardless of whether they are roasted or raw—are typically not soaked and dried before they are made into butter.

To properly prepare nuts, pour raw nuts into a glass or ceramic bowl. Cover the nuts with filtered water.

Allow the nuts to soak overnight—with the exception of cashews, which should only soak for 2 to 3 hours, and macadamia nuts, which cannot be soaked, lest they disintegrate into mush.

After soaking, drain and rinse the nuts well.

Spread onto cookie sheets lined with parchment paper and dry in the oven on the lowest setting overnight or until dried and crunchy. Alternatively, spread onto dehydrator sheets and dry. The setting recommended for nuts is the same amount of time as soaking.

Now your nuts are ready to be made into butter, ground into flour, or eaten by the handful.

≈ Honor Sacred Foods: Eggs, Liver, Organ Meats, Bone Broth, and Seafood ↶

Before you turn the page in repulsion, did you know that most traditional cultures strove to eat the whole animal whenever possible? This was not only to stretch their meals, but also because they knew that the organs of animals are rich in important fat-soluble vitamins, minerals, and other nutrients. In Chinese medicine, this is as close as we get to replenishing Jing through food.

We're not suggesting that you sit down with a knife, fork, and a whole buffalo, but we do want to shed light on the fact that there's more to a chicken than boneless, skinless breasts, and there's more to beef than a filet mignon.

Eggs are one of the easiest sacred foods to incorporate into your diet. They contain all nine essential protein-building amino acids. A whole egg contains about 5 grams of fat, which will aid you in absorbing the eggs' fat-soluble vitamins A, K, E, D, and B-complex as well as minerals such as iron, phosphorus, potassium, and calcium. Eggs also contain choline, which is an important component found in every living cell.

Eat at least two whole eggs per day as part of your nutrient-dense fertility diet. Seek out eggs from hens that have been raised on pasture, eating the natural forage-fed diet of chickens: grasses, seeds, and bugs. If you cannot source pasture-raised eggs, your next best option is free-range organic. Cage-free and organic eggs not labeled free-range should be avoided as they are inferior quality.

✴ HOW TO MAKE PERFECT HARD-BOILED EGGS ✴

Boil enough filtered water to cover as many eggs as you plan to boil. Once your water is boiling, use a spoon to gently drop in eggs so that they do not crack. Allow them to boil for exactly 10 minutes for slightly soft or 12 minutes for completely cooked through.

IF YOU'D LIKE TO SAVE YOUR EGGS FOR LATER: Drain the hot water from the pot, cover the eggs in cold water, and add a scoop of ice. When they're cool, remove from the water and store in the fridge until you're ready to eat.

IF YOU'D LIKE TO EAT YOUR EGGS RIGHT AWAY: Drain the hot water from the pot and bounce the eggs in the pot so that the shells crack. Cover the eggs in cold water and add a scoop of ice. After about two minutes, drain, peel your eggs, and enjoy.

MINI-FRITTATAS

We know you're busy, but that's no excuse to skip the most important meal of the day. These mini-frittatas are super easy to throw together over the weekend and enjoy for a last-minute breakfast (or lunch) on the go. This recipe features spinach and feta cheese, but you can easily swap for your favorite frittata fillers—ham and Swiss, bacon and Cheddar, or a medley of seasonal veggies.

Butter or olive oil, for greasing
4 cups (120 g) spinach leaves
1 medium onion
3 cloves of garlic
1 ounce (28 g) Parmesan cheese
8 eggs
1½ teaspoons sea salt
½ teaspoon black pepper
¼ cup (60 ml) cream
2 tablespoons (28 ml) olive oil
4 ounces (115 g) feta cheese (optional)

Preheat the oven to 400°F (200°C, or gas mark 6). Grease a muffin tin with butter or olive oil. Chop spinach and onion. Mince the garlic. Shred the Parmesan cheese.

In a large mixing bowl, whisk together the eggs, salt, pepper, cream, and Parmesan cheese; set aside.

Over medium heat, sauté the onions in the olive oil until translucent. Add the garlic and cook another minute. Add the spinach and cook until just wilted and bright green in color.

Spread the spinach mixture evenly on the bottom of the muffin cups. Pour the egg mixture evenly over the spinach and onions. Crumble the feta, if using, over the top of the frittata. Bake for 10 to 12 minutes or until the frittata is nice and golden and the eggs are set.

Carefully remove the pan from the oven and let the mini-frittatas cool for several minutes before serving. When cool, store leftovers in the fridge in a covered airtight container. Throughout the week, these mini-frittatas can be easily heated in a toaster oven or even enjoyed cold.

Yield: 12 mini-frittatas

BACON TOMATO QUICHE
WITH CAULIFLOWER CRUST

Quiche is a wonderfully versatile food. It's great for breakfast, lunch, or even a light dinner served with a simple green salad. This version features an unusual cauliflower crust, which keeps the dish grain-free and only adds to the deliciousness.

As with the mini-frittatas, the options for the filling are endless, so if you're not in the mood for tomato and bacon—follow your taste buds and get creative. Quiche also makes for a good grab-and-go breakfast for mornings when time is limited.

FOR THE CRUST:

1 tablespoon (14 g) butter

½ a head of cauliflower

1 egg

1 cup (150 g) grated mozzarella cheese

¼ cup (25 g) grated Parmesan cheese

1 teaspoon oregano

1 teaspoon sea salt

½ teaspoon garlic powder

½ teaspoon onion powder

½ teaspoon black pepper

FOR THE FILLING:

4 eggs

1 cup (235 ml) cream

1 teaspoon sea salt

¼ teaspoon freshly ground black pepper

½ teaspoon paprika

8 ounces (225 g) bacon

1 large ripe tomato or 1 cup (150 g) cherry or grape tomatoes

4 green onions

8 ounces (225 g) Cheddar cheese

To make the crust: Preheat the oven to 450°F (230°C, or gas mark 8). Grease the bottom of a pie dish or similar sized baking dish with butter.

Break the cauliflower into florets. Using the s-blade with your food processor, pulse the cauliflower florets until they are the consistency of rice. Steam the cauliflower in a covered saucepan until cooked but not mushy (no need to add water). Measure out 1 cup (165 g) of cooked "riced" cauliflower for this recipe and freeze the rest in a resealable plastic bag for a later meal.

Combine the cooled cauliflower, egg, mozzarella, Parmesan, oregano, sea salt, garlic powder, onion powder, and black pepper in a small bowl. Using your hands, spread the raw "dough" into a thin layer on the bottom of your greased baking dish.

Bake for 20 to 25 minutes or until the crust is uniformly browned. Remove from oven and set aside.

Reduce oven temperature to 350°F (180°C, or gas mark 4).

To make the filling: In a large bowl, beat the eggs and then mix in the cream, salt, pepper, and paprika.

Cut the bacon into slivers. In a large skillet, cook the bacon until just crisp. Set aside. When slightly cool, drain the bacon fat through a fine-mesh strainer into a clean mason jar and save to use as cooking fat.

Slice the tomato and dice the green onions. Shred the cheese. Evenly distribute the bacon, tomatoes, green onions, and cheese in the prebaked crust. Pour the egg mixture over top.

Bake the quiche for 30 minutes or until set. Serve immediately or warm later in the oven.

Yield: 6 to 8 servings

CREAMY EGG DROP SOUP

This soup is perfect for breakfast, which may sound funny, but why not? This simple recipe combines homemade broth, eggs, and a touch of Asian flavors that can turn any naysayer in a soup-for-breakfast convert.

- **1 quart (946 ml) homemade chicken broth**
- **2 whole eggs**
- **2 egg yolks**
- **1 teaspoon toasted sesame oil**
- **1 to 2 tablespoons (15 to 28 ml) fish sauce to taste**
- **2 green onions**

Heat the broth in a saucepan to a simmer. Remove from heat.

In a separate bowl, beat the eggs and extra egg yolks.

Using a ladle or measuring cup, slowly pour the broth into the eggs, whisking the entire time until combined.

Dice the green onions. Stir in the sesame oil and fish sauce to taste, garnish with green onions, and serve.

If reheating, do so over gentle heat. If the eggs congeal, use an immersion blender (or standing blender if you don't have one) to bring the consistency back to its silken state.

Yield: 4 servings

MAGICAL CHILI

This chili is not only magically delicious, but the disguised organs pack a nutrient-dense punch. Below is a double batch so you can freeze half and have a quick meal for later.

2 large onions

4 cloves of garlic

2 tablespoons (28 g) butter, lard, or tallow

1 tablespoon (15 g) sea salt

2 tablespoons (15 g) chili powder

2 teaspoons oregano

1 teaspoon cinnamon

1 teaspoon ground cumin

½ teaspoon allspice

½ pound (225 g) mushrooms

2 or 3 sweet peppers (bell or Italian, any color)

2 pounds (900 g) grass-fed ground beef

1 pound (455 g) heart and/or liver from beef or chicken

1 can (28 ounces, or 785 ml) diced tomatoes

4 ounces (115 g) tomato paste

1 quart (946 ml) beef or chicken stock

Sea salt to taste

Sour cream or strained yogurt, for garnish

Chop the onions and mince the garlic. In a large stockpot, sauté the onions in the butter and 1 tablespoon (15 g) sea salt. Add garlic, chili powder, oregano, cinnamon, cumin, and allspice. Chop the mushrooms and peppers. When the onions are translucent, add the mushrooms and peppers.

If the liver and/or heart are whole, run through a food processor with an s-blade until ground.

Add the ground meat and organs to the sautéing vegetable. Brown the meat over medium heat. Break it up finely with a wooden spoon. Add the tomatoes, tomato paste, and stock. Adjust seasoning to your preference.

Serve immediately topped with sour cream or allow to simmer for several hours to combine the flavors. When cool, freeze half of this recipe for a later meal.

Yield: 4 to 6 servings per batch

CALIFORNIA BURGERS

We just love real food makeovers, especially when something as fun as a burger gets to star in your healthy, nutrient-dense diet. With grass-fed beef and the secret addition of liver, you can indulge with joy. Top with grass-fed cheese, avocado—heck—even bacon for extra fertility-promoting fats.

> **⅛ to ¼ pound (57 to 115 g) liver**
> **1 pound (455 g) ground beef**
> **1 teaspoon sea salt**
> **1 teaspoon garlic powder**
> **1 teaspoon onion powder**
> **½ teaspoon black pepper**
> **1 tablespoon (14 g) bacon fat**
> **4 ounces (115 g) Cheddar cheese (optional)**
> **Sourdough buns (optional)**
> **1 avocado**
> **Cultured Ketchup (page 87)**

Add the liver to a food processor and blend until smooth.

In a large bowl, add the ground liver, ground beef, salt, garlic powder, onion powder, and black pepper. Using clean hands, combine the ingredients well and form into 4 patties.

Heat the fat in a skillet on high heat and cook the burgers for 3 minutes on the first side. Flip and cook for 3 minutes on the other side. Meanwhile, slice the cheese, if using. Add the cheese and cook for 1 more minute until medium rare, longer if you prefer your burgers well done.

Serve on a toasted bun, topped with sliced avocado and cultured ketchup.

Yield: 4 burgers

LIVER

So what makes liver so wonderful? According to the Weston A. Price Foundation, it contains more nutrients, gram for gram, than any other food and is also:

* An excellent source of high-quality protein
* Nature's most concentrated source of vitamin A
* Abundant in all the B vitamins, particularly vitamin B_{12}
* One of our best sources of folate, the nonsynthetic form of folic acid
* A highly usable form of iron
* Our best source of copper (and also contains trace elements of zinc and chromium)
* An unidentified antifatigue factor
* High in CoQ_{10}, a nutrient that is especially important for cardiovascular function
* A good source of purines, nitrogen-containing compounds that serve as precursors for DNA and RNA

* HOW TO MAKE HOMEMADE LIVER "PILLS" *

Feel a little like Sam I Am when we talk about liver? Not in a house, not with a mouse. . . . What about if you could just take a pill? Would you take your liver then?

These homemade liver "pills" are the best solution to eating liver without *eating* liver.

Start with 1 pound (455 g) of liver from healthy pasture-raised beef, lamb, bison, or chicken.

Keep the liver frozen for a minimum of 14 days to destroy any pathogens. If you're purchasing fresh liver, make the pills and then freeze for 14 days before consuming.

When ready to make the liver pills, defrost the liver, rinse, and pat dry. With a sharp knife, coarsely chop into ¼- to ½-inch (6 mm to 1.3 cm) pieces.

Line a lipped, freezer-safe dish with parchment paper. Spread the liver pieces over the paper, and lay a piece of plastic wrap over top and freeze for several hours until solid.

When completely solid, transfer the frozen liver "pills" into an airtight container and store in the freezer. Swallow a couple of frozen liver pills with every meal. Avoid taking liver pills with milk or other dairy as the calcium in the milk can block iron absorption.

MONICA'S CHICKEN LIVER PÂTÉ

The French know what's up when it comes to nutrient-dense food—especially ones that you can spread all over freshly baked bread. If you don't eat grains—pâté is great on cucumber slices or seed crackers, too. This recipe is the creation of Monica Ford, who runs our favorite real food delivery service, Real Food Devotee.

3 tablespoons (42 g) bacon drippings	½ cup (64 g) arrowroot
1 small shallot	2¼ (14 g) teaspoons salt
6 cloves of garlic	1 teaspoon black pepper
3 cups (210 g) cremini mushrooms	½ teaspoon freshly grated nutmeg
2 tablespoons (5 g) fresh thyme	½ teaspoon ground allspice
⅓ cup (80 ml) cognac or other brandy	8 to 10 tablespoons (112 to 140 g)
1 pound (455 g) chicken livers	unsalted butter or ghee
10 egg yolks	Several fresh bay or sage leaves
2 cups (475 ml) cream	(optional)

Preheat the oven to 350°F (180°C, or gas mark 4).

Melt the bacon drippings in a heavy skillet over medium heat.

Finely chop the shallots. Mince the garlic. Slice the mushrooms. Add the shallots, stirring occasionally, until softened, about 4 minutes. Add the garlic, mushrooms, and thyme. Cook, stirring, about 4 minutes. Remove from the heat carefully add the cognac (use caution; if the cognac ignites, shake the skillet), and then boil until reduced to a thick consistency with little liquid.

Allow the mixture to cool—don't skip this step! Transfer the glorious-smelling mixture to a blender or food processor. Add the livers and yolks, and then purée until smooth. Add the cream, arrowroot, salt, pepper, nutmeg, and allspice and blend until combined. Pour the pâté into a butter-greased terrine, skimming off any foam.

Make a water bath by putting your filled terrine in a larger baking dish and adding enough boiling water to reach halfway up the side of the smaller terrine. Place in the oven and bake until the pâté is just set and a small sharp knife inserted in center comes out clean, about 50 minutes.

Melt the butter in a small saucepan over low heat, and then remove from the heat and let stand for 2 minutes. Spoon enough butter over the pâté to cover its surface. A thick layer will provide a nice seal, which will increase your pâté's shelf life.

Chill the pâté completely, about 4 hours. Freeze or store in the refrigerator depending on when you plan to enjoy it. Bring to room temperature about 1 hour before serving.

Yield: 8 servings

ORGAN MEATS

Other organ meats besides liver also have nutrient-dense merits. Beef heart, for instance, has more highly concentrated protein than regular muscle meats and is very high in CoQ_{10} (an antioxidant that may contribute to ovarian health), B vitamins, iron, and folate—nutrients essential for healthy conception and pregnancy. The texture of heart can be a bit tough, but stewing or braising allows the meat to become nice and tender.

Kidneys from pasture-raised animals are high in potassium, B_{12}, iron, zinc, folate, and vitamins A and D. The traditional British steak-and-kidney pie is the most well-known dish utilizing this organ, but kidneys from veal, lamb, pork, and beef can all be braised, roasted, sautéed, and even grilled.

More and more restaurants are popping up featuring "nose to tail" cuisine, including more common dishes such as liver pâté and pork belly sandwiches as well as dishes less familiar to the Western palate such as tripe, brains, and sweetbreads. When sourced from properly raised animals, these "alternative" meats can all be considered fertility super-foods. Put on your adventurous spirit and enjoy!

BONES

If you've been mostly eating lean chicken breasts and steak, you might have forgotten that meat actually comes with bones. In Chinese medicine, the bones are ruled by the Kidney meridian/Water element—the same energy that governs our reproductive potential. Eat meat on and from the bone whenever possible; try bone marrow and consume bone broth regularly.

BASIC ROAST CHICKEN AND ROOT VEGGIE PURÉE

One of the simplest ways to incorporate bones into your diet is by roasting a whole chicken and eating the meat off the bones. This recipe includes roasted potatoes and carrots, but feel free to substitute any root veggies with thin skin of your choice to save time by not having to peel them (yams, turnips, radishes, rutabaga, etc.). As a bonus, you'll have chicken bones for making broth when the meal is done and any meat is removed for leftovers.

1 whole chicken	A sprig of rosemary
1 large onion	½ cup (112 g) butter, lard, or
4 small potatoes	coconut oil
2 carrots	Unrefined sea salt
½ of a lemon	Freshly cracked black pepper
1 head of garlic	

If using frozen chicken, the night before, remove the chicken from freezer and defrost in a sink or large bowl of cool water.

About 1½ hours before dinner, preheat the oven to 375°F (190°C, or gas mark 5). Remove the chicken from the package, remove the giblet bag from the chicken cavity, rinse well, and pat dry. Slice the onion and cube the potatoes and carrots.

Place the onion and root veggies in a baking dish and set the chicken atop with the legs under the chicken. Stuff lemon, garlic, and rosemary into the chicken cavity. Rub ¼ cup (55 g) softened butter over chicken skin. Sprinkle generously with salt and pepper.

Bake for 30 minutes. Using tongs and/or potholders, gently flip the chicken so that the legs are up. Sprinkle salt and pepper on the flip side of the chicken and bake for another 30 minutes or until the skin is nicely browned and crisp. Remove from the oven and check that the root veggies are soft when a fork is inserted. If not, gently remove the chicken to a serving platter and place the veggies in the oven for another 20 to 30 minutes or until tender.

When the veggies are soft, transfer them to a food processor with the pan juices. Add the remaining ¼ cup (55 g) butter and purée until smooth.

Yield: 4 servings

BONE BROTH

The name "bone broth" sounds medieval, like something modern folks simply don't eat. But more and more, people are turning back to stock made with the bones of chicken, beef, fish, and so on for both superior culinary flavors and old-fashioned healing properties.

Every chef and foodie knows the key to a good soup or sauce is the stock. Bone broth tastes far superior to any canned or carton varieties, but beyond flavor, it's also far more nutritious. Homemade broth is loaded with minerals, gelatin, and glycosamino-glycans (which include substances such as chondroitin and glucosamine, keratin and hyaluronic acid, and more). These nutrients benefit skin, teeth, bones, hair, nails, and joints.

Bone broth is also a digestive elixir that helps heal the gut lining—a big benefit for those who suffer from digestive problems, food allergies, and nervous system conditions including anxiety and depression. When the digestion is working optimally, inflammation is quelled throughout the body. The digestive benefits of bone broth support fertility because, as we have seen, strong digestion is central to good health.

Bone broth is also a rich source of minerals including calcium, magnesium, phosphorus, silicon, sulfur, and other trace minerals that are vital for creating a healthy new life. Ancient South American proverbs tell that broth will even decrease the pain of childbirth. Because bone broth is easily digestible, these minerals are absorbed by the body.

Aim to drink a minimum of 1 to 3 cups (235 to 700 ml) of bone broth per day, either by the mugful or used in soup, stew, to cook grains, or in other recipes. Beyond that, use your beautiful broth as the base for soups and sauces, to cook rice or quinoa, or in any recipe that calls for stock.

BEGINNER'S CHICKEN BONE BROTH

So you want the health benefits of bone broth, but you haven't cooked much beyond boiling water for spaghetti and heating up sauce or grilling a chicken breast in a pan? No problem. Even the most remedial beginners can master a basic chicken bone broth. This version is for squeamish beginners, folks who "don't cook," and anyone short on time. You know those rotisserie chickens they sell at grocery stores? Perfectly cooked whole chicken, ready for you to take home for dinner = real food for no effort = brilliant.

If you are a true beginner, you probably buy the roasted chicken, pick off the meat, and toss the bones in the . . . WAIT! Don't throw the bones away. This is where the fun begins. Follow this method for quick and easy broth.

> **1 rotisserie chicken (preferably organic and free-range)**
> **Filtered water**
> **1 tablespoon (15 ml) apple cider vinegar**
> **Onion and/or onion peels, carrots, and celery (optional)**

Eat your store-bought rotisserie chicken. Place the remaining "frame" of the chicken (the bones, skin, and cartilaginous bits) into a slow cooker or stockpot.

Cover the bones with water, adding 1 tablespoon (15 ml) apple cider vinegar per chicken frame. Top with the lid and cook on low for a minimum of 6 hours up to 24 hours or until the bones crumble when pinched.

Carefully strain the broth through a fine-mesh metal sieve and discard the bones. Use the broth immediately, store in the fridge for about a week, or freeze for future use in ice cube trays for quick defrosting. If saving for later, consider concentrating the broth by simmering it until it is half of its volume to save on space in your fridge or freezer.

Yield: Approximately 1 gallon (3.8 L)

POACHED WHOLE CHICKEN AND BONE BROTH

If you regularly roast your own chickens at home, you can follow the instructions on page 103. If you have a whole chicken to work with, poaching it in a slow cooker yields more consistently tender meat than roasting. Poaching also makes it easier to completely remove the meat from the bones to eat in sandwiches, salads, and stir-fries.

1 whole chicken, including giblets
Filtered water
1 tablespoon (15 ml) apple cider vinegar
Onion and/or onion peels, carrots, and celery (optional)

Remove the (defrosted or fresh) chicken from its packaging, and remove any giblet bag inside the cavity. Rinse and place the chicken and giblets in the slow cooker. Add filtered water to just cover the chicken. Turn the slow cooker to low and cook for 3 to 4 hours (depending on the size of the chicken and the heat of your pot) until the chicken is just cooked (no longer pink).

Remove the chicken and place it in a separate bowl until cooled. Cut or shred the meat from the bones. Put the bones, skin, and other bits back into the slow cooker with the broth and apple cider vinegar, cover, and continue simmering on low for 6 to 12 hours.

Strain the broth through a fine-mesh metal sieve and discard the bones. Use the broth immediately, store in the fridge for about a week, or freeze for future use.

Yield: Approximately 1 gallon (3.8 L)

✳ EXTRA CREDIT: ADDING FEET, NECKS, HEADS, AND MORE ✳

Today, in a boneless-skinless-chicken-breast culture, we are trained to think that lean muscle meat is the best source of animal protein. Au contraire! It is indeed the offal, the bones, and the fat of properly raised animals that provide us with important fat-soluble vitamins and microminerals that are lacking in white meat.

When you receive the heads and feet from your farmer, they most likely have already been cleaned, so there is nothing more to do other than gingerly or exuberantly dump them in your stockpot.

BIELER'S BROTH

Originally created by Henry Bieler, M.D., "for fasting, for energy, and for overall health," our version is made with chicken broth to help tonify "reproductive essence." Try eating it with breakfast for a nourishing and cleansing start to the day.

4 medium zucchini
1 pound (455 g) string beans
2 stalks of celery
1 to 2 bunches of parsley
Fresh herbs such as thyme or tarragon (optional)
1 quart (946 ml) Beginner's Chicken Bone Broth or
    Poached Whole Chicken and Bone Broth (page 104)
Sea salt to taste

Slice the zucchini, remove the ends from the string beans, chop the celery, and remove the stems from the parsley. Tie the fresh herbs (not including fresh parsley) together with kitchen string.

Add the zucchini, string beans, celery, tied herbs, and chicken broth to a large saucepan. Turn heat to high and cook until the veggies are bright green. Remove from the heat and add the parsley.

Using an immersion blender, blend into a soup, stopping at your preferred consistency. Season with sea salt to taste.

Yield: 1 quart (946 ml)

BEEF BONE BROTH

Ask your farmer or butcher for bones for making stock. Be sure to get some joint and knuckle bones, which will impart gelatin to your finished products. Apple cider vinegar is essential to leach minerals out of the bones.

> **5 to 8 pounds (2.3 to 3.6 kg) bones from pastured beef,**
>   **bison, pork, or lamb**
> **1 head of garlic**
> **2 to 3 tablespoons (28 to 42 g) fat such as coconut oil, lard,**
>   **or tallow, for roasting**
> **Filtered water**
> **2 tablespoons (28 ml) apple cider vinegar**
> **2 or 3 bay leaves (optional)**

Rinse and clean the bones with water; pat dry and rub with fat. Roast the bones with the garlic at 400°F (200°C, or gas mark 6) for 45 minutes to 1 hour, turning once, until they are well browned. This ensures a good flavor in your resulting stock.

Add the roasted bones and the pan scrapings to a big pot, cover with filtered water, and bring to a boil. Once boiling, add the vinegar, bay leaves, and garlic. Turn down the heat and simmer covered for several hours, ideally up to 24 hours. Throughout the simmering process, skim off any scum and add water as needed to keep bones covered.

When the stock has finished simmering, allow it to cool. Filter through a fine-mesh strainer and refrigerate until chilled. Once chilled, the stock should set like gelatin (but don't worry if it doesn't), and the fat should rise to the top. Pick off the fat and reserve it for cooking.

Scoop out the gelled stock and reheat to serve straight or to use for a recipe. Store extra in the fridge for a week or so or freeze in PVC/BPA-free plastic freezer bags, mason jars, or ice cube trays.

Yield: Approximately 1 gallon (3.8 L)

SIMPLE VEGGIE SOUP

This is the most simple and versatile soup, and you can whip it together in no time. Feel free to use whatever veggies and herbs that are seasonal and you have on hand and be sure to season generously with sea salt and freshly ground pepper to allow the flavors of the homemade stock and veggies to shine.

> 1 onion
> 3 tablespoons (42 g) butter or coconut oil
> 2 carrots
> 2 stalks celery
> 1 large potato
> 1 medium zucchini
> 1 small handful of green beans
> 3 cloves of garlic
> 1 quart (946 ml) chicken stock
> 2 sprigs of thyme
> ¼ of a lemon
> Sea salt and freshly ground pepper
> ½ cup (115 g) yogurt, for garnish (optional)

Trim and roughly chop the onion. In a large saucepan over medium-high heat, melt the butter and sauté the onions with a big pinch of sea salt until they begin to soften.

Trim and roughly chop the carrots, celery, potato, zucchini, and green beans. Mince the garlic. When the onion is softened, add the veggies and garlic to the saucepan with the chicken stock and thyme.

Turn up the heat to high and bring to a boil. Reduce the heat and simmer until the potatoes are soft when mashed with a fork.

Remove from the heat. Remove the thyme. Using an immersion blender, blend until smooth. Season with the juice from ¼ of a lemon, salt, and ground pepper to taste. Garnish with an optional swirl of yogurt.

Yield: 2 quarts (1.9 L)

POMEGRANATE GELATIN

You may remember J-E-L-L-O fondly from your childhood—from shapely molds with suspended fruit cocktail to a bowlful topped with Cool Whip.

Even Kraft Jell-O is a relatively simple food containing "sugar, gelatin, adipic acid (for tartness), contains less than 2% of artificial flavor, disodium phosphate and sodium citrate (control acidity), fumaric acid (for tartness), red 40, blue 1." But our version is made with gelatin from grass-fed beef (such as Great Lakes brand) and fresh juice.

We use 1 cup (235 ml) liquid to 1 tablespoon gelatin. If you prefer a more spoon-able, jellylike result (especially good topped with raw whipped cream or crème fraîche), use less gelatin. The dessert will taste less sweet than your original juice, so if you prefer a sweeter result, stir in a touch of raw honey before cooling to set. Experiment with stir-ring in some fresh berries or a swirl of raw cream before chilling.

4 cups (946 ml) fresh pomegranate juice, divided
4 tablespoons (55 g) Great Lakes gelatin

Add the gelatin to 2 cups (475 ml) cold juice and stir. Set aside.

Bring the remaining 2 cups (475 ml) juice to a boil and then add to the gelatin/juice mixture. Stir to dissolve the gelatin and pour into a shallow pan. Place in the fridge to cool. When completely gelled, cut into cubes (or used a fun shaped cookie cutter) and enjoy!

Yield: 6 to 8 servings

✳ MARROW ✳

The only thing that's more of a Jing tonic than bones and bone broth is marrow. Marrow is the fatty substance within the bones and you may be surprised by how delicious it tastes. More and more often we're seeing bone marrow appear on restaurant menus, and once you taste bone marrow spread on crusty bread, it may appear in your dreams, too.

According to Ramiel Nagel, author of *Cure Tooth Decay*, eating marrow even on occasion will strengthen your body's resilience against cavities because it helps rejuvenate bone and promote bone growth. We would take marrow over cake any day, and that says a lot.

ROASTED BONE MARROW

If you haven't already discovered your love for meat butter, you're in for a treat. Many restaurants now serve marrow on their fancy menus, but this recipe is super easy to make at home and will save you a bundle so you can eat it as often as your heart desires.

> **6 center-cut marrow bones**
> **3 tablespoons (45 ml) olive oil, divided**
> **1 slice of sourdough toast**
> **2 cloves of garlic**
> **1 tablespoon (6 g) lemon zest**
> **1 tablespoon (4 g) finely chopped parsley**
> **Sea salt and coarse black pepper**
> **1 sourdough baguette**

Preheat the oven to 450°F (230°C, or gas mark 8). Rinse the bones and pat dry. Place the bones vertically on a baking tray lined with parchment paper and brush them with 1 tablespoon (15 ml) olive oil.

Break the toast into small pieces and pulse in a food processor to make bread crumbs. Mince the garlic. Mix the bread crumbs, garlic, lemon zest, parsley, and remaining 2 tablespoons (28 ml) olive oil. Season with a generous pinch of sea salt and grind of pepper. Lightly toss.

Spoon the crumb mixture on top of each bone and roast until the marrow is soft throughout, yet not so soft it melts away. Start checking (by inserting a thin skewer) at 10 minutes for smaller bones and at 15 to 20 minutes for larger bones. Serve with a hot sourdough baguette and small spoons for scooping.

Yield: 3 to 4 servings

SEAFOOD

Most thriving traditional cultures revered seafood, often going out of their way to trade for fish if they did not live near the coast. Wild-caught, oily fish such as salmon and black cod are of particular value for fertility. But the real stars are actually seafood that can be consumed whole: sardines and anchovies, mollusks, and fish roe.

While caviar is considered a rich man's food, other fish eggs can be remarkably affordable—especially when you consider the nutrient-dense punch they pack. A single ounce (28 g) of roe contains 8 grams of protein and 873 milligrams of omega-3 fats and 54 percent of the RDA for vitamin B_{12}. If you are concerned about the yuck factor, a tiny portion goes a long way, and the salty/sour flavor enhances most savory dishes including dips, salads, sandwiches, and sushi.

Aside from fish roe, mollusks—oysters, clams, mussels, and scallops—are one of the easiest and most efficient ways to benefit from eating the whole animal because they are small and relatively easy to gather. Mollusks are rich in zinc, iron, selenium, and other trace minerals; fat-soluble vitamins A and D; and the long-chain omega-3 fatty acids DHA and EPA.

For optimal nutrition, eat fresh seafood two to four times per week, with a focus on fish roe, mollusks, shellfish, salmon, sardines, and anchovies.

✳ THE OYSTER-APHRODISIAC CONNECTION ✳

The old wives' tale that oysters act as an aphrodisiac was recently backed up by research when a team of American and Italian scientists discovered that beyond zinc, shellfish (oysters in particular) are high in rare amino acids that trigger the increased levels of sex hormones in both men and women that help to improve libido.

CONCERNED ABOUT MERCURY IN SEAFOOD?

There is quite a bit of concern in the media and among health practitioners and consumers alike about the risk of mercury toxicity from eating too much seafood.

Mercury toxicity is definitely something you want to avoid if you are trying to conceive, both for the success of getting pregnant and the health of your future children. That said, there is often a missing piece to the mercury conversation that makes it much less scary.

Selenium is an essential nutrient that counteracts the effects of mercury by binding to it and making a new substance that then allows mercury to pass out of the body without binding to human tissue and creating harm. Because of the strong affinity that selenium has for mercury, as long as selenium is present in higher quantities than mercury, you are safe to consume fish, even if it contains the harmful element.

The U.S. Environmental Protection Agency has proposed a new measure of seafood safety called the Selenium Health Benefit Value (SeHBV) that takes the protective role of selenium into account. Lucky for fish lovers, many of the fish that are high in mercury are also higher in selenium—with shark and swordfish being the only two fish known to be consistently low in selenium.

If you're still concerned about mercury toxicity in fish, we recommend including a selenium supplement when you are eating fish that may be higher in mercury. With the protection of selenium—either from the fish itself or in a supplement—you can enjoy the culinary delights and nutritional benefits of seafood without worry.

CEVICHE AND COCONUT OIL TORTILLA CHIPS

Ceviche is a delicious way to eat seafood, bursting with tangy goodness while keeping all of the nutrients intact. Rest assured that ceviche uses the acidity of citrus to denature the protein in a manner similar to cooking. As always, use the freshest fish you can find.

FOR THE CEVICHE:

2 pounds (900 g) very fresh white-fleshed ocean fish (halibut, snapper, tilapia, etc.)

1 cup (235 ml) freshly squeezed lime juice (about 7 limes)

½ cup (120 ml) freshly squeezed lemon juice (about 3 lemons)

½ cup (120 ml) freshly squeezed orange juice (about 3 small oranges)

½ of a jalapeño pepper

1 red bell pepper

¼ of a red onion

3 cloves of garlic

1 teaspoon raw honey

¼ cup (4 g) chopped fresh cilantro

2 teaspoons sea salt, plus more to taste

2 avocados

FOR THE TORTILLA CHIPS:

1 dozen sprouted corn tortillas

2 to 3 cups (450 to 675 g) coconut oil (depending on the size of your pan; you want at least 1 inch [2.5 cm] of oil)

To make the ceviche: Dice the fish. Remove the seeds and pith from the jalapeño; wear gloves to avoid burning your skin. Include some seeds if you prefer more heat. Finely dice the bell pepper and mince the onion and garlic.

Place the fish in a glass dish with the citrus juices, jalapeño, bell pepper, onions, garlic, and sea salt. Toss to coat. Cover and refrigerate for at least 3 to 4 hours (preferably overnight) stirring occasionally.

To make the tortilla chips: Using a cleaver or pizza cutter, cut the tortillas into eighths. Place a mesh strainer above a large bowl.

Heat the fat over medium-high heat in a large skillet until shimmering. Add the tortillas in a single layer. Fry until lightly golden and crispy and then transfer to mesh strainer. (Think fast-food french fry draining!) Continue frying in batches, taking care to avoid spatter from the hot oil. Season with sea salt to taste.

Before serving, dice the avocado and stir into the chilled ceviche with the honey and cilantro. Season with additional sea salt and lime to your taste and serve with the tortilla chips.

Yield: 6 servings

MUSSELS IN COCONUT RED CURRY SAUCE

It may seem intimidating to make something like mussels at home, but we promise it's easy and well worth it. The combination of the seafood, coconut milk, and curry spices makes a delicious, comforting, and fertility-boosting meal.

> 1½ pounds (680 g) mussels
> 1 can (14 ounces, or 390 g) unsweetened coconut milk
> 2 cloves of garlic
> 1 stalk of lemongrass
> 1 lime
> 2 tablespoons (30 g) red curry paste
> 1 teaspoon sucanat
> 1 tablespoon (15 ml) fish sauce
> 3 tablespoons (7.5 g) chopped fresh basil

Scrub and debeard the mussels in cool water, discarding any that don't close to the touch. Shake the coconut milk well before opening the can. Mince the garlic and cut the center white of the lemongrass into 1-inch (2.5 cm) pieces before crushing. Cut the lime in half. Juice one half and cut the other half into wedges.

In a wok or stockpot, combine a few table spoonfuls (45 to 60 ml) of the coconut milk with the garlic, lemongrass, curry paste, and sucanat over medium heat. Stir for 5 minutes or until smooth and fragrant. Stir in the remaining coconut milk, ½ cup (120 ml) filtered water, fish sauce, and juice of half the lime. Raise the heat to high and add the mussels. Cover and cook until the mussels open, 4 to 6 minutes.

Transfer the mussels to a large shallow serving bowl, discarding any that are unopened. Ladle the broth over the mussels, garnish with basil and lime wedges, and serve with steamed rice.

Yield: 4 servings

MUSTARD-CRUSTED SALMON

If you haven't perfected the skill of cooking fish at home, give this recipe a try for a quick and satisfying meal any day of the week.

1 pound (455 g) baby red potatoes

3 tablespoons (42 g) butter or coconut oil, melted

2 teaspoons sea salt

Freshly ground pepper

2 slices of sourdough toast

¼ cup (60 g) Dijon mustard

1 tablespoon (9 g) dried mustard

1½ pounds (680 g) wild-caught salmon fillets (6 ounces, or 170 g, per person)

Preheat the oven to 375°F (190°C, or gas mark 5). Cut the potatoes into quarters. In a large roasting pan, toss the potatoes with the melted fat and season with sea salt and pepper. Spread the potatoes evenly in the pan and roast for about 20 minutes.

While the potatoes are roasting, break the cooled toast into 1-inch (2.5 cm) chunks. In a small food processor, pulse the toast to form coarse bread crumbs. Set aside.

Combine the mustards in a small bowl and coat the nonskin side of the salmon fillets with the mustard mixture. Then sprinkle evenly with bread crumbs, pressing gently to form a crust.

Remove the potatoes from the oven and nestle the salmon fillets in the roasting pan with the potatoes.

Bake for an additional 15 minutes or until the fish is just cooked through and the topping is beginning to brown. Remove from the oven and serve with a seasonal green salad.

Yield: 4 servings

~ Clear Excess with Cleansing Foods ~

While they're all the rage in modern health circles, generally speaking, cleanses are not as healthy as they're cracked up to be. Most cleansing regimens are either too extreme (lemon water and cayenne pepper for days on end) or just a fancy way to get you to spend a fortune on supplements. And at the end of a cleanse, most people go back to life as usual, creating a yo-yo extreme in diet that does not typically yield lasting beneficial results and can wreak havoc on your metabolism.

That said, it *is* wise for nearly everyone to incorporate *some* cleansing into their diets, both by regularly consuming greens and vegetables and occasionally having an extended period of eating *relatively* lighter than your typical day-to-day.

For the average person, an appropriate time to switch to a more cleansing diet is in the spring because it is the season of growth and renewal. Springtime also correlates to the Liver/Gallbladder system, which fits perfectly with the idea of cleaning house, since the Liver is the primary organ for detoxification in our bodies. Decreasing heavy meat and starch consumption is seasonally appropriate in the springtime. You may even find you crave these foods less with the change of season toward warmer weather and longer days, so instead of beef barley stew, you may choose to have a mixed green salad with seared fish.

For those who suffer from "excess" heat and toxicity as discussed on page 70, cleansing foods should be part of a weekly or even daily focus. For those women taking fertility medicines, hydrating and cleansing foods may be helpful to restore balance after a cycle of medication. With the addition of some simple fresh vegetable juices to your diet, you can easily incorporate a gentle cleanse that is ideal when recovering from a course of medication, including the time between egg retrieval and embryo transfer for women undergoing IVF.

The amount of cleansing foods you eat should be based on how they feel in your body. Do your symptoms clear after several days with a focus on lighter, cleansing foods? Do you feel more energetic and experience more mental clarity when you eat this way? These are signs that the cleansing foods are appropriate. While intense detox reactions and "healing crises" are not unheard of, stimulating your body to dump toxins should not be your goal—lighter, gentler feelings of cleansing are much preferred.

By adding green veggies, light vegetable soups, and other foods and drinks that have a cleansing effect, you lighten the load for the digestive system, which allows the nervous system to operate more smoothly, as well. Following are some simple ways to cleanse wisely.

Start your body's cleansing process by including more greens—especially dark leafy greens, including bok choy, kale, chard, spinach, and collards. Young, leafy greens such as baby lettuces or dandelion leaves and seasonal veggies such as asparagus and peas are ideal for cleansing, too. You can also add some cleansing, cooling, and refreshing herbs and spices to your favorite light meals, including green onions, dill, cilantro, oregano, green garlic, and fennel.

GREEN SOUP

This green soup is the perfect way to incorporate a cleansing element to your diet. It also tastes surprisingly fantastic and is filling and hearty. Though delicious at any time of the day, this soup makes a great breakfast food. Try it topped with grilled salmon or a small spoonful of leftover quinoa or rice for a more substantial meal. This recipe is a serving for one because it's best to make this fresh to order.

¼ onion
1 to 2 large handfuls of kale
¼ cup (33 g) frozen peas
1 cup (235 ml) homemade bone broth or filtered water
1 small handful of dried wakame seaweed
1 tablespoon (16 g) unpasteurized miso
Juice of ¼ lemon
1 tablespoon (15 g) tahini paste (optional)
Unpasteurized soy sauce to taste (optional)

Chop the onion. Wash and chop the kale. Place the onions and peas in a medium saucepan, cover with bone broth or filtered water, and bring to a boil.

Add the kale and dried seaweed. Steam/blanch briefly until the greens are emerald in color. Add the miso and lemon juice. Use an immersion blender or countertop blender to purée the contents of the pot (including liquid).

Spoon into bowls, top with optional tahini and soy sauce, and serve immediately.

Yield: 1 serving

WILTED DANDELION GREENS WITH LEMON AND FETA

This is a simple side dish that can add a cleansing element to any meal, from a breakfast of scrambled eggs to a side dish for a roast. You can typically find dandelion greens at major health food stores year-round, but in many areas, this common weed grows wild and you can forage for it yourself (just don't pick from polluted areas on the side of the road).

On their own, dandelion greens are very bitter greens (great for addressing heat and "dampness"). When sour lemon and salty feta cheese are added, the bitterness of the green is tempered. You can also add small handfuls of chopped dandelion to salad, stir-fries, and soups to incorporate the cleansing benefits into other meals.

1 bunch of dandelion greens
Juice of ¼ lemon
Olive oil or butter
4 tablespoons (38 g) feta cheese

Wash and finely chop the dandelion greens. Place the greens directly in a pan (no need to add extra water). Cover and steam for a quick minute or two until the greens are bright green. Remove from the heat. Rinse briefly under cool water to slow the cooking process. Toss to remove water.

Douse with lemon juice and olive oil. Top with crumbled feta cheese and serve.

Yield: 1 to 2 servings

EAT RAW WITH MODERATION

While we all benefit from the enzyme content of raw veggies, aim to eat no more than 20 percent of your veggies in raw form because raw, cold foods can further damage weakened digestion. Instead, lightly steam veggies and toss with a bit of coconut oil, butter, lard, ghee, or olive oil. Fat helps your body assimilate minerals from vegetables, while cooking makes them more digestible.

DRINK YOURSELF CLEAN

Water, tea, and fresh juices are great ways to aid your body's cleansing process. Green tea, fresh mint, chrysanthemum, red clover, and dandelion teas help to clear excess heat and toxicity. You can also find natural detox or cleansing teas at most health food stores. Sip these cool or hot.

You can also try adding a pinch of sea salt and some sliced lemon and orange to your drinking water for extra-refreshing, extra-hydrating mineral water.

FERTILITY TEA

Herbal teas are a great way to support reproductive health while both gently cleansing and hydrating. The herbs listed in this tea blend are some of the most commonly used for supporting fertility. Feel free to modify to suit your taste.

Some suggested ingredients are as follows:

- **RED RASPBERRY LEAF**—Tonifies the uterus, supports pregnancy, and is high in minerals
- **ROSE HIPS OR ROSEBUDS**—Relieves stress and supports the immune system
- **OAT STRAW**—Soothes the nervous system, and is rich in calcium, silica, and B vitamins
- **MINT**—Cools the body and relieves stress

Combine 4 to 5 tablespoons (24 to 30 g) of these herbs (your choice of combination) in a quart-sized (946 ml) mason jar, cover with boiled and slightly cooled water (about 30 seconds off boil), and steep for 15 to 20 minutes. Feel free to add a squeeze of lemon and/or a touch of raw honey.

ELECTROLYTE DRINKS

Staying hydrated isn't just for athletes! Electrolytes, which are made up of various salts, provide your body with the ability to send impulses across your cell membranes. That's fancy talk for "they send signals that tell your body what to do."

Without electrolytes, your cells are like a train car with no conductor, and over time, a crash is more than likely.

Store-bought electrolyte drinks are not generally recommended because they are filled with artificial colors, sweeteners, and other toxic junk. Not to worry, though, making electrolyte drinks for yourself is easier than you might think; see the recipes on page 120.

COCONUT WATER

Coconut water has made its way into the limelight recently, and we approve. Coconut water, the clear liquid found inside young (green) coconuts, contains more potassium than four bananas and is loaded with B vitamins, minerals, and electrolytes. Athletes often use it for post-workout replenishment, sometimes with a pinch of sea salt or Himalayan pink salt for extra repletion.

We recommend coconut water in its raw form, ideally from a coconut you've cracked yourself, or from a health food store that sells it in an unheated, untreated form.

BONE BROTH

Season to taste with your favorite salt and sip your way to rehydration with this super-food electrolyte beverage.

TOO MUCH LIQUID

We know you've heard that you should drink 8 to 10 glasses of water per day—or half your body weight in ounces. While some folks definitely need to drink more water and fluids, the health-nut, water-guzzling craze does not apply to everyone. Remember that most fresh foods contain water, and drinking too much can disrupt your electrolyte balance, actually interfering with healthy metabolism by diluting digestive juices.

To assess your fluid consumption and urinary output, listen to your body:

* Are you thirsty throughout the day? Do you have dark, scanty pee? Do you get headaches, which are made better by drinking water? You may need to drink more.
* Are you constantly drinking water and peeing clear? You may need to back off your fluid consumption.

EASY ELECTROLYTE TEA

Just about anything can become an electrolyte solution by adding some salt and sugar to the mix. Choose a favorite herbal tea and add a pinch of Himalayan pink salt or Celtic sea salt, citrus juice, and a healthy sweetener such as honey or maple syrup using the proportions given here.

1 liter (about 1 quart) purified water
1 teaspoon salt
Juice from 2 lemons or limes
Herbal tea of your choice (mint, chamomile, rooibos, etc.)
Honey or maple syrup to taste

Brew the herbal tea in 1L (1 quart) of purified water. Then add a pinch of salt, lemon juice, and a drizzle of honey.

Yield: 1 liter (about 1 quart)

EASY HOMEMADE THIRST QUENCHER

This has all of the benefits of the common sports drink minus the neon colors and other weird stuff.

½ cup (120 ml) freshly squeezed orange juice
¼ cup (60 ml) lemon or lime juice
2 cups (475 ml) purified water
⅛ teaspoon Himalayan or Celtic sea salt
Honey or maple syrup to taste (about 2 tablespoons, or 40 g)

Mix together the juices, water, salt, and honey. Serve cold.

Yield: 2¾ cups (650 ml)

∼ "But I'm Vegetarian! What About ME?" ∼

We're going to be honest. When it comes to supporting fertility and pregnancy, a vegetarian diet has its challenges—especially so if you're vegan.

We have worked with countless vegan and vegetarian women who found their plant-based food choices were no longer adequate when they were trying to conceive or to maintain a healthy pregnancy and postpartum recovery. It's not to say it can't be done, but extra care is needed to make sure you get it right.

While most criticism of a vegetarian diet is around whether you're getting enough protein, in fact, protein is not usually the biggest worry since most health-conscious herbivores know they need to piece together enough of this nutrient from grains, beans, nuts, and more.

The bigger concern is getting enough healthy fat, cholesterol, and fat-soluble vitamins—especially D, A, and K_2. While it's commonly believed that these nutrients (and others) can be supplied from plant sources (vitamin A in carrots, zinc in grains, and vitamin D in fortified orange juice, for example) these nutrients are far more useful to the body from animal sources, such as vitamin A in liver, zinc in oysters, and vitamin D from fermented cod liver oil and pastured lard.

GUIDELINES FOR VEGETARIANS
WHO WANT TO GET PREGNANT

If consuming animal foods for the sake of optimizing your fertility is off the table, then use the following guidelines to maximize the benefits of your vegetarian diet:

1. Aim for an ovo-lacto diet, which is the best vegetarian option if you are trying to optimize fertility. Dairy and eggs will provide you with essential fat, cholesterol, fat-soluble vitamins, and protein. Also, if you are open to eating fish and/or other seafood, now's the time to do so.

2. Consume coconut (oil, cream, milk, and meat from coconuts), avocados, and palm oil from sustainable sources (which *guarantee* that they protect the habitats of orangutan) daily.

3. Properly prepare your grains, legumes, seeds, and nuts by souring, soaking, or sprouting. This will ensure that your body has access to their full nutritional profile and that antinutrients do not block absorption of minerals from the rest of your food.

4. Only consume *fermented* soy, such as tempeh, miso, and unpasteurized soy sauce.

5. Consume cultured foods including fermented vegetables, condiments, and drinks daily.

6. Consider a vitamin D supplement (see page 134 to determine whether you're getting enough).

7. Eat natto (fermented soybeans) or take a vitamin K_2 supplement (see page 138 to learn more about this important and seldom discussed nutrient).

8. Watch your vitamin A intake. Vitamin A is a tough one. We don't recommend supplementing with synthetic vitamin A due to its potential toxicity when taken in this form. As we'll discuss more on page 137, the conversion of beta-carotene to true vitamin A is often not adequate, so those committed to a vegetarian diet may find themselves lacking in this important nutrient for baby-making. Aside from supplementing with cod liver oil or liver pills, the next best option is to eat orange foods (such as carrots, sweet potatoes, and papaya) that contain carotenes.

9. Take vitamin B_{12} supplements. Vitamin B_{12} is necessary to produce red blood cells and prevent anemia. Found almost exclusively in animal products, it is impossible to get enough B_{12} on a vegan diet alone. Vitamin B_{12} deficiency may go undetected in vegans because the vegan diet is rich in folate, which may mask deficiency in vitamin B_{12} until severe problems occur.

10. Take an omega-3 supplement. If you are willing to take a fermented cod liver oil supplement, it will provide you with omega-3s, plus fat-soluble vitamins D and A that one cannot get from plant sources. We recommend the brand Green Pasture for its sustainable, well-sourced fermented cod liver oil. Vegetarian food options for omega-3s include flax, hemp, walnut, and algae. These sources contain the fatty acid ALA, which ideally can convert to DHA and EPA; however, studies show that the human body does not convert this very well. The best vegetarian option is from microalgae, which can provide all three essential fatty acids (DHA, EPA, and ALA).

Unless you're extremely deficient, it's possible that, once pregnant, your baby will get all of the nutrients he or she needs regardless of what you eat. Still, if you're not consuming the right foods, the placenta will demand calcium from *your* bones, fatty acids from *your* brain, and other nutrients it needs from *your* body, leaving you feeling less than wonderful as your baby grows and in need of serious repletion after baby is born.

By following these guidelines, however, you can optimize your vegetarian diet for fertility, pregnancy, and beyond—both for the health of your child and yourself.

✳ THE CHEAT SHEET FOR FEEDING YOUR FERTILITY ✳

Here's a quick recap. Mark this page so you can refer back to this summary whenever you need a refresher. Or better yet, make a copy and paste it to your fridge.

EAT WHAT YOUR GREAT-GREAT-GRANDMOTHER ATE.
. . . or someone else's g-g-grandma if you prefer their style of cuisine! This means home-cooked meals, seasonal produce, meat, fish, raw dairy from the right sources (pasture-based, sustainably raised), and cultured foods.

DITCH THE JUNK.
Purge your pantry and stop eating and buying processed foods today. When you give yourself permission to eat well-sourced butter, bacon, cream, and more, suddenly packaged food becomes much less exciting.

EAT MORE FAT.
Include some saturated fats with every meal—butter, cream, coconut oil, bacon, etc. Olive, seed, and nut oils are good, but they can go rancid easily and should not be heated to high temperatures. DON'T consume new-fangled, refined vegetable oils such as canola, corn, or soybean oil.

INCLUDE CULTURED FOODS.
Eat cultured foods and drinks such as yogurt, kefir, sauerkraut, kimchi, kombucha, and fermented condiments every day to cultivate healthy digestion, central to good health.

PROPERLY PREPARE GRAINS, LEGUMES, AND NUTS.
If grain, bean, and nut consumption is not negatively contributing to your health, be sure to consume these foods after they have been properly prepared through soaking, sprouting, or souring.

HONOR SACRED JING FOODS.
Homemade soups made with bone broth, chicken liver pâté, fish eggs, bone marrow, oysters—these are just a few of the sacred foods that can profoundly enhance your reproductive potential. Don't overlook these foods just because they seem too odd for your palate. Read more about the health benefits of these Jing foods on page 68.

EAT FOR YOUR CHINESE MEDICINE CONSTITUTION.

Food is your best medicine. While all couples who are trying to conceive should focus on Jing foods, choose appropriate foods to address your own personal imbalances from the Chinese medicine perspective you've learned in this book.

GET INSPIRED.

Maybe it's indulging in raw oysters or perhaps it's beginning the day with fried eggs. Don't get overwhelmed thinking you have to adopt a real food lifestyle all at once. Start with something that sounds good to you. Your body will begin to thank you for eating nutrient-dense food and ask for more.

EAT WITH JOY!

How we eat is just as important as what we eat, so eat regular meals, be present while you are munching, and enjoy every bite.

Chapter 9

Vitamins and Supplements for Fertility

WE LIVE IN A FOOD SCIENCE CULTURE where it's encouraged to choose your food by reading labels, counting calories, and tallying fiber grams and vitamin values. Modern folks count on multivitamins and superfood shakes to supply them with the best nutrition possible.

We believe that for most people, it is completely possible to receive adequate, excellent nutrition through diet alone. While some supplementation may be necessary for a particular individual in a particular circumstance, it is best to try to meet nutritional needs through food first, then choose targeted supplements to fill in any gaps or deficiencies.

∽ Why Food Is the Best Prenatal Nutrition ∾

In our modern Western world, prospective mothers and pregnant women are sent to the pharmacy with a prescription for synthetic supplements, which are often difficult for the body to digest and absorb.

Prenatal vitamins are like an insurance policy to (hopefully) avoid deformities and abnormalities in your child. Taking care to eat the right foods will take you beyond disaster prevention and help pave the way for faster conception, a smoother pregnancy, and a child with radiant health.

This approach may seem scary and even unsafe to many women who are accustomed to our "health by pill" culture, but consider that the U.S. Recommended Daily Allowances of nutrients *are* based on what has been determined to be an ideal human diet. Logically, then, we should be able to get these nutrients from food.

Here are the conventional nutritional recommendations for pregnancy outlined by Dr. Mikio Nihira on WebMD.com (in the first three columns) and the equivalent real food suggested servings (in the last column).

While macronutrients (fat, protein, and carbohydrates) are not included on this chart, they are all essential to your prenatal nutrition. In particular, saturated fat and cholesterol (from animal sources) allow for the proper absorption and assimilation of

Nutrient	Benefits	Pregnancy RDA	Real Food Sources
Calcium	This builds strong, dense bones in mother and child and may help prevent high blood pressure in pregnant women.	1,000 mg; don't exceed 2,500 mg	1 cup plain full-fat yogurt (415 mg); 1 cup whole milk (about 300 mg); 1 ounce Cheddar cheese (204 mg).
Choline	This helps prevent neural tube defects and enhances brain development.	450 mg; don't exceed 3,500 mg	1 egg (272 mg); 3 ounces pork tenderloin (103 mg), ground beef (83 mg), salmon (65 mg), or chicken (65 mg).
DHA	Boosts baby's brain development and vision. Improves sperm and egg quality. Reduces inflammation in all cells of the body.	300 mg	3 ounces oily fish (740 mg); fermented cod liver oil.
Folic Acid	Helps protect against neural tube defects during the first 30 days of pregnancy and possibly cleft palate; reduces anemia in mom and helps prevent early miscarriage and premature delivery.	600 micrograms	No real food contains folic acid—it is synthetic only. Instead, consume liver a few times a week for folate (one chicken liver = 254 mg). 1 cup spinach, broccoli, collards, asparagus (60 mg); garbanzo beans (1 cup = 282 mg).
Iron	As part of red blood cells, iron ferries oxygen, wards off anemia in mom, and helps prevent premature delivery.	27 mg; don't exceed 45 mg.	3 ounces clams, oysters, or mussels (12 mg); 3 ounces beef (3 mg), lamb (2 mg), or chicken liver (11 mg).
Vitamin B₆	Assists in the production of protein for new cells; bolsters the immune system; and participates in red blood cell formation.	1.9 mg	1 cup chickpeas (1.1 mg); 3.5 ounces beef liver (1 mg); 3 ounces tuna (0.9 mg).
Vitamin B₁₂	Assists in red blood cell production and helps the body use fat and carbohydrates for energy.	2.6 micrograms	3 ounces clams, mussels, or oysters (42 micrograms); salmon (5 micrograms); rainbow trout (4 micrograms); tuna (3 micrograms); or beef (2 micrograms).
Vitamin D	Promotes calcium absorption from food and its deposition into mom's and baby's bones and teeth.	4,000 IU	1 teaspoon fermented cod liver oil (1,950 IU); lard from pastured pigs; oysters (270 IU for about 6); fish roe (up to 17,000 IU per tablespoon).
Zinc	Critical for cell growth and repair; energy production; and brain development.	11 mg; don't exceed 40 mg.	3 ounces oysters (76 mg), beef (9 mg), crab (5 mg), or pork (4 mg); or 1 cup full-fat yogurt (2 mg).

vitamins and minerals and are essential for nearly every function in the body. If you are consuming adequate saturated fat, it's likely you are also eating enough high-quality protein (as most saturated fats—with the exception of coconut and sustainable palm oils—are in meat, fish, eggs, and dairy).

Also missing from the chart on the previous page is vitamin A, due to its alleged toxicity. When it is a component of food (as opposed to synthetic vitamins), vitamin A is not toxic and is indeed essential to supporting your fertility and growing a healthy baby.

The chart at the right outlines how to match and exceed the nutritional requirements of a prenatal vitamin through food sources. These recommendations are in line with those of the Weston A. Price Foundation.

WAPF PRENATAL RECOMMENDATIONS

Fertility Foods	Recommended Servings
Full-Fat Dairy	4 cups total of whole, raw milk daily plus an additional 4 tablespoons (55 g) butter from grass-fed cow; 2 ounces (155 g) raw cheese = 1 cup milk
Eggs	Aim for 2 per day
Seafood	2 to 4 times per week plus Fermented cod liver oil to supply 20,000 IU vitamin A and 2,000 IU vitamin D
Liver	3 to 4 ounces (85 to 115 g) 1 or 2 times per week plus Fermented cod liver oil to supply 20,000 IU vitamin A and 2,000 IU vitamin D
Bone Broth	At least 1 to 3 cups (235 to 700 ml) per day
Beef or Lamb	Daily
Coconut Oil	2 tablespoons (28 g) daily
Cultured Food	Aim for some (at least a tablespoon or two) with every meal
Fresh Fruit and Vegetables	Some with each meal
Properly Prepared Grains	Decide based on your ability to digest them.

Essential Nutrients	Sources
Saturated fat • Cholesterol Vitamin K_2 • Vitamin A	Source from pasture-raised cows, preferably NOT pasteurized or homogenized, but at minimum: use organic and full-fat. This includes whole milk, cream, yogurt, kefir, buttermilk, sour cream, crème fraîche, ice cream, and cheese.
Saturated fat • Cholesterol Omega-3 fatty acids • Vitamin A • Vitamin E • Choline	Eggs from pasture-raised hens are ideal. If not available, always choose free-range organic eggs.
Saturated fat • Cholesterol • Omega-3 fatty acids • Vitamin D • Vitamin B_{12} • Trace minerals • (zinc, copper, selenium, and iron)—in shellfish	• Oily fish: salmon, sardines, herring, anchovies, and trout • Fish roe • Shellfish: Mussels, clams, oysters (raw from reliable sources or cooked), lobster, crab, and prawns (especially when consumed whole). • Fermented cod liver oil
Saturated fat • Cholesterol • Vitamin A • Omega-3 fatty acids • Folate • Vitamin B_{12} • Pantothenic acid • Riboflavin • Niacin	• Liver from healthy pasture-raised animals • Fermented cod liver oil
Calcium • Magnesium • Phosphorus • Gelatin • Glucosamine • Chondroitin • Silicon • Sulfur • Trace minerals	Use homemade bone broth from poultry, beef, lamb, or fish bones. Include the feet, joints, and the heads of chicken and fish if they are available. Store-bought stock is not an acceptable substitute.
Saturated fat	With the fat
Saturated fat	Use in cooking or smoothies.
Probiotics	Yogurt, crème fraîche, kefir, traditionally fermented sauerkraut, kimchi, cultured condiments, and kombucha
Various vitamins, minerals, and enzymes	Choose produce that is local, seasonal, and organic whenever possible. On average, no more than 20 percent should be eaten raw. Consume with some saturated fat for best nutrient absorption.
Carbohydrates, various vitamins and minerals	Whenever you eat grains Proper preparation of grains will reduce antinutrients. See page 89 for an explanation on how to choose or properly prepare grains, legumes, and nuts.

Take a good look at what you eat in a typical week and write it down. If your diet is not consistently predictable, keep a food journal for at least a week or two to get an adequate idea of everything you put in your mouth—food and drink. Next, compare your diet with the recommendations with the second chart here:

* What are you already eating each day/week? Keep doing that.
* What would be easy to incorporate? Start doing that now.
* What are you willing to try?
* What are you simply not willing or able to consume (whether because of personal taste, allergies, or accessibility)?

Based on these discoveries, you now can start to get an idea of if and how you need to supplement your diet. If you would rather turn a blind eye to food-as-nutrition, the next best option is to take a food-based prenatal vitamin and eat a diet rich in high-quality saturated fat and cholesterol; synthetic vitamins alone are not adequate preparation for healthy conception, pregnancy, birth, or baby.

∼ Choosing Supplements ∼

In a perfect world, all women trying to conceive would eat a complete, nutrient-dense diet for at least three months before conception and all the way through nursing. That said, we understand that it's not realistic to expect every person reading this book will be ready or capable of committing to getting all her necessary nutrition through real food. With that in mind, we will include both food and the best supplement alternatives as we go through our nutritional recommendations. In all cases, it's important to determine if and how your diet is lacking and then make up the rest with supplements that are primarily food-based (as opposed to synthetic).

In the next section, we will cover each of the following supplements in full detail:

* Omega-3s—Recommended for everyone trying to conceive
* Fat-soluble vitamins (D, A, K_2)—Should be adequate with real food diet, but some supplementation may be necessary
* Probiotics—For those with digestive or immune system concerns, or anyone who doesn't consume cultured foods daily
* B vitamins—Supplementation often needed for vegetarians and those under extreme stress
* Minerals—Should be adequate with real food diet, but occasionally supplementation is necessary
* Amino acid therapy—For those with mood disorders or extreme food cravings
* Additional antioxidants—For those with extreme toxic overload

* A food-based prenatal vitamin—For those severely lacking in nutrition from food
* Chinese herbs—Your practitioner will work with you to customize herbal formulas to support your cycle and address imbalances specific to you.

OMEGA-3S

Fish oil is one of the best ways to get essential omega-3 fatty acids and is the only supplement that we recommend for nearly every patient we see. Omega-3s are essential to all human beings and in particular are important for fertility and pregnancy to:
* Improve hormone functioning
* Increase blood flow to reproductive organs
* Soothe the nervous system to address the effects of stress on fertility
* Improve sperm and egg quality when taken for a minimum of three months
* Prevent erectile dysfunction
* Promote the healthy development of the fetus's brain
* Reduce the risk of pregnancy-induced hypertension
* Reduce the risk of gestational diabetes
* Reduce inflammation associated with pain and discomfort
* Manage stress to keep mom and baby healthy

You can find omega-3s nearly everywhere these days—in the news, in your eggs, even in your trail mix. There's no question that this nutrient plays a crucial role in human health, but choosing the right omega-3 sources can be mind-boggling. Following is what we recommend to our patients.

FISH OIL
When it comes to choosing fish oil, quality is important. You want to be sure to choose a brand that tests for mercury and other contamination; uses minimal processing to keep the oils as virgin as possible; and chooses fish from a sustainable source.

COD LIVER OIL
Fish oil is an excellent source of omega-3s, but cod liver oil has the added benefits of being naturally rich in the fat-soluble vitamins D and A. The problem with most commercially available cod liver oil brands is that they undergo a deodorization process by which most of the naturally occurring vitamins are removed. The vitamins A and D are then added back in with too little vitamin D in ratio to vitamin A, which can lead to toxicity.

Because of this common practice, many health experts warn against cod liver oil, but in fact, they should be warning against *processed* cod liver oil. In its natural form, cod liver oil is a perfect natural supplement for vitamins A and D. According to Dr. John Cannell, founder of the Vitamin D Council, the safe and ideal ratio is approximately 1:5. Currently, the only minimally processed cod liver oil on the market is Green Pasture Fermented Cod Liver Oil (FCLO), which is the fish oil recommended by the Weston A. Price Foundation.

Proponents of FCLO say that because it is a fermented food, the body can assimilate its nutrients with more ease and efficacy. Other folks debate the necessity of fermenting cod liver oil at all, saying that oil does not ferment. Personally, we do not take sides about the fermentation either way but *do* appreciate that FCLO provides vitamin A and D in the correct ratios. This is especially important if you are not getting these fat-soluble vitamins otherwise (typically through sunshine and regular consumption of liver).

KRILL OIL

Krill are small crustaceans that live in cold ocean areas. Krill oil is a rich source of omega-3s, and it also contains a natural antioxidant called astaxanthin and undisclosed amounts of vitamins A, E, and D. There are several more advantages to krill oil over other fish oils. Krill is:

* Easier to digest—doesn't produce a fishy aftertaste
* More potent as an antioxidant
* Less likely to be contaminated with toxins because krill is a tiny animal
* Protect against skin damage from UV exposure because it contains astaxanthin

* HOW MUCH FERMENTED COD LIVER OIL DO YOU NEED? *

One teaspoon of high-vitamin fermented cod liver oil contains 9,500 IU vitamin A and 1,950 IU vitamin D, a ratio of about 5:1. The Weston A. Price Foundation recommends the following dosages for fermented cod liver oil:
• Pregnant and nursing women and those trying to conceive: 2 teaspoons or 20 capsules, providing 19,000 IU vitamin A and 3,900 IU vitamin D
• Children over 12 years and adults: 1 teaspoon or 10 capsules, providing 9,500 IU vitamin A and 1,950 IU vitamin D

The downsides to krill are that it does not contain vitamins A or D in adequate amounts, and it can be fairly expensive. However, during the summer months if you are getting enough sun exposure for vitamin D as well as eating liver regularly, krill may be a good choice.

Whichever fish oil you choose, be sure to choose oils that are cold-pressed, as this technique preserves nutritional value and purity of oils. Cold-pressing methods yield less oil than higher heat methods, resulting in pricier oils but also higher quality and optimum nutritional value.

FINAL NOTES ON DHA IN FOODS AND VITAMINS

There are different types of omega-3 fatty acids—DHA, EPA, and ALA. DHA and EPA (found in fish, grass-fed beef, etc.) are the fatty acids that your body can readily utilize. ALA (found in flax, hemp, and other plant-based sources) needs to be converted by the body to DHA—and this is not always done sufficiently.

You may notice that grocery store foods advertise DHA in yogurt, cereal, trail mix, and eggs. As of this writing, the FDA is not required to label type and amount of omega-3s; so despite these claims, these foods are most likely supplemented with ALA, and the amounts may not match claims. We recommend that you simply opt for omega-3s from high-quality fish sources.

Also, prescription prenatal vitamins often come in a packet and contain a few DHA capsules to cover your omega-3 needs. As with supplements in general, we'd prefer that, rather than singling out DHA, you choose a separate fish oil supplement of known origin and quality.

VITAMIN D

Until recently, vitamin D has been an underappreciated nutrient, but in the last several years, research as well as empirical evidence has been showing that vitamin D is essential for fertility and overall good health.

According to a 2012 review in the *European Journal of Endocrinology,* vitamin D:

* Improves in vitro fertilization (IVF) outcomes
* Helps resolve endometriosis and polycystic ovary syndrome (PCOS) in women
* Supports progesterone and estrogen levels in women, which regulate menstrual cycles and improve the likelihood of successful conception
* Is essential for the healthy development of sperm cells
* Helps maintain semen quality and sperm count
* Increases levels of testosterone in men, which may boost libido

While it is believed that the human body synthesizes vitamin D best through regular sun exposure, even with your best efforts, it is difficult to get enough D-generating sunshine during the winter months in most parts of the Northern Hemisphere. Human beings used to spend much more time outdoors; our ancestors spent the majority of daylight hours hunting and gathering and, more recently, plowing the fields all day in the sun.

These days, even those of us who are sun-lovers spend a large portion of our days working indoors and slathering ourselves with sunscreen when outside. Fortified dietary sources (such as conventional milk and gummy vitamins) contain only a tiny fraction of the D needed for optimal health.

Vitamin deficiencies often go undetected until health problems and/or fertility issues occur. The only way to accurately determine your level is by blood test. Cannell and other holistic-minded experts recommend 50 to 90 ng/ml as a normal range of D_3 blood levels. While it is optimal to get vitamin D through sunshine and food-based sources, using a vitamin D_3 supplement may be essential if your blood levels are significantly low.

THE THREE BEST WAYS TO GET VITAMIN D

Sun on our skin is the most natural source of vitamin D, but lifestyles, climate, and environmental factors can make this challenging. Here are your options when it comes to getting enough of the sunshine vitamin.

Get vitamin D via sun exposure. Keep the following in mind if you want to raise your vitamin D levels with sun exposure:

* At least 40 percent of the body's skin should be exposed to the sun.

* Light-skinned people need approximately 10 to 20 minutes of sun exposure daily, while very dark-skinned people may need up to 90 to 120 minutes daily. Estimate one-quarter of the time it would normally take to burn.
* Washing exposed areas with soap or swimming in chlorine removes natural skin oils necessary for vitamin D generation. Instead, rinse with water and wash only "essential" areas with soap.
* Avoid using sunscreens during therapeutic exposure.
* During winter months, additional foods rich in vitamin D may be necessary.

Get vitamin D through food. Following are some top sources:
* **FERMENTED COD LIVER OIL**—Read more about this supplement on page 132.
* **LARD FROM HEALTHY FORAGING PIGS**—This may come as a surprise: After cod liver oil, lard is the second-best source of vitamin D. The key is getting lard from pigs that haven't been factory-raised, have spent time outdoors in sunshine, and have eaten a healthy diet. Good-quality bacon and bacon grease is a great gateway into the wonderful world of lard. See page 79 for a tutorial on rendering your own.
* **OYSTERS**—Six oysters contain an estimated 270 IU of vitamin D, but keep in mind that your body utilizes nutrients from food far more easily than from supplements.
* **FISH ROE**—You know those tiny orange things you get with sushi? The ones with a salty flavor that bursts in your mouth? It's called fish roe—and it's packed with D. A recent WAPF-funded analysis by UBE Laboratories showed a single tablespoon (15 g) of roe contained 17,000 IU of vitamin D.

Supplement with vitamin D3. While the only way to accurately determine your vitamin D level is by blood test, the recommended dosage to maintain normal D_3 levels is estimated to be 35 IU/pound of body weight. If you take adequate cold-pressed cod liver oil and/or get sufficient sun exposure, you will not need to supplement unless your blood levels are low.

Here's how to determine if and how much vitamin D supplementation you need:
* After two months of taking recommended dosages and/or getting vitamin D from sunshine or food sources, have a 25-hydroxy-vitamin D blood test done, which tests for D_3 (cholecalciferol). Your health practitioner can administer this test or you can order a home kit online.
* Adjust your dose and retest as needed so your 25(OH)D level is between 60 and 90 ng/ml year-round.

If you need to supplement, be sure to take vitamin D_3, which is the type your body needs (not D_2). A tincture in olive or coconut oil of 2,000 IU/drop is our preferred way to supplement when necessary. Supplementing with vitamin D_3 is generally considered safe despite it being a fat-soluble vitamin because the levels necessary for overdose are incredibly high. Though there are no reports of vitamin D toxicity in humans, based on animal studies, it would take 176,000,000 IU of vitamin D to kill a 110-pound (50 kg) person, or you would need to be taking approximately 40,000 IU daily over time. Toxicity is simply not a concern in levels below 10,000 IU daily.

Finally, be sure you're consuming an adequate amount of calcium- and magnesium-rich foods while supplementing, because without these nutrients in sufficient quantities, vitamin D will cause calcium to be withdrawn from your bones. Though vitamin D is currently the darling of the vitamin industry, as with all other nutrients we strongly suggest that you aim to get yours through natural means—this means sun and vitamin D foods—with supplements as a last choice.

✳ HOW NOT TO GET VITAMIN D ✳

It's important to note that many "trusted" sources of vitamins and minerals fall short in both quality and dosages. Some commonly relied-upon, inadequate sources of vitamin D include the following:

- **MULTIVITAMINS**—Multivitamins simply do not contain vitamin D in adequate levels. Many of these pills and gummies also don't contain the right type of vitamin D (D_3 as opposed to D_2).
- **BREAKFAST CEREAL**—There are many reasons to skip cereal, but when it comes to vitamin D, similar to multivitamins, it's not going to provide you with anything close to the dosage of vitamin D you need.
- **FORTIFIED MILK (OR ORANGE JUICE)**—The milk and juice industries have most of us believing our drinks have vitamin D covered. They don't, for the same reasons stated above.
- **COD LIVER OIL THAT DOES NOT HAVE VITAMINS A AND D IN THE CORRECT PROPORTION**—Spend the extra effort on sourcing fermented cod liver oil. Or alternatively, choose a high-quality fish oil and supplement with foods rich in vitamins A and D.
- **TANNING BEDS**—Individuals with poor gut absorption or seasonal affective disorder can benefit from making vitamin D during winter months with the aid of tanning beds' UVB rays. However, nature did not intend for humans to sit in an electrically charged box. In most cases, the risks of x-ray and EMF (electromagnetic fields) in tanning beds outweigh the benefits.

VITAMIN A (FROM FOOD ONLY)

True vitamin A (found in animal sources) is one of several fat-soluble activators that are necessary for the assimilation of minerals in the diet. Vitamin A is important for eye health and, according to Sally Fallon Morell, vitamin A is the "concert master for a developing fetus"—something you don't want to miss if you're trying to conceive a healthy baby.

WHY NOT JUST EAT CARROTS AND CALL IT A DAY?

There are two forms of vitamin A: preformed vitamin A (also known as retinol) and carotene.

Basically, animal sources such as cod liver oil, liver, eggs, whole milk, cream, and butter contain true, preformed vitamin A. Carotene is a precursor found in deep green and yellow or orange vegetables, which, under ideal circumstances, your body can convert into vitamin A in the upper intestinal tract.

Unfortunately, you would need to eat a ridiculously large quantity of carotene-rich fruits and vegetables to meet your daily requirement. Carotene is also not well converted in most infants and children or people who:

* Eat a low-fat diet
* Consume excessive iron (especially from "fortified" cereals and other grain products)
* Consume a diet high in polyunsaturated fats
* Suffer from diabetes, hypothyroidism, pancreatic disease, or digestive issues including diarrhea or celiac disease
* Engage in strenuous physical exercise
* Consume excessive alcohol

LET'S CLEAR UP THE CONFUSION ABOUT VITAMIN A AND TOXICITY

There is some major conflicting information regarding the toxicity of vitamin A, and as a result, the recommended dosages conflict as well.

A 1995 study from the *New England Journal of Medicine*, "Teratogenicity of High Vitamin A Intake," concluded that preformed vitamin A taken in excess of 10,000 IU per day by pregnant women was linked to birth defects. This single study received a great deal of attention, and consequently, the FDA currently recommends that pregnant women get their vitamin A from foods containing beta-carotene and no more than 5,000 IU of preformed vitamin A (if any) per day.

However, according to a recent edition of the *Merck Manual* (a well-respected medical textbook), only two fatalities of acute vitamin A toxicity have ever been reported when "within a few hours of ingesting several million units of vitamin A in polar bear or seal liver, arctic explorers developed drowsiness, irritability, headache, and vomiting, with subsequent peeling of the skin. Mega-vitamin tablets containing vitamin A have occasionally induced acute toxicity when taken for a long time, however, chronic toxicity usually develops after doses of >100,000IU/day have been taken for months. Birth defects have been reported in the children of women using 13-cis-retinoic acid [commonly known as Accutane] for skin conditions during pregnancy."

From her thorough article "Vitamin A Saga," Sally Fallon Morell reports, "The US Recommended Daily Allowance of vitamin A is currently 5,000 IU per day (and may possibly be lowered to 2500 IU per day). From the work of Weston Price we can assume that the amount of vitamin A found in primitive diets was about 50,000 IU per day."

No wonder folks are so confused, with such conflicting information from experts. To be on the safe side, we recommend that you rely on true vitamin A from food sources rather than a synthetic supplement.

Remember, while carotene can provide vitamin A through conversion, it is not a reliable source. There is no need to worry if you eat some squash or carrots (or even a prenatal vitamin) with your eggs and liver because carotene is not known to cause toxicity in large quantities or in combination with preformed vitamin A.

VITAMIN K_2

Vitamin K_2 is a little-known but extremely important fat-soluble vitamin. We classically think of vitamin K for its role in blood clotting; however, this task is accomplished by vitamin K_1, which is found in leafy green plants.

Vitamin K_2 on the other hand, is primarily found in dairy and liver from animals raised on grassy, sunny pastures as well as some fermented foods. Vitamin K_2 plays a

---

✳ BEST SOURCES OF TRUE VITAMIN A ✳

- **FERMENTED COD LIVER OIL** (see page 132 for recommended dosages)
- **LIVER FROM PASTURE-RAISED, HEALTHY ANIMALS**—1 or 2 times per week
- **LIVER PILLS**—either desiccated in capsules or frozen homemade "pills" (recipe on page 48)
- **RAW, UNPASTEURIZED MILK OR CREAM**—2 to 8 ounces (60 to 235 ml) of milk per day for pregnant or nursing moms
- **EGGS FROM HENS RAISED ON PASTURE**—2 or more per day

key role in being distributed properly to bones and teeth and preventing calcium from being deposited into soft tissue such as blood vessels and kidneys. Vitamin K_2 also aids in the synthesis of important fats involved in brain metabolism. When it comes to baby-making, vitamin K_2 is essential to ensure the proper growth and development of a fetus as well as maintaining good health for the mother-to-be.

WHICH FOODS CONTAIN VITAMIN K2?

An official U.S. Recommended Daily Allowance for vitamin K_2 has not been established at this time, but some holistic-minded practitioners recommend aiming for 100 mcg/day. According to a study in the *Journal of Agriculture and Food Chemistry*, the top 10 sources of vitamin K_2 are:

* Natto—1103.4 mcg K_2/100G*
* Goose liver pâté—369.0 mcg K_2/100G (100 g = 3.53 ounces)
* Hard cheeses—76.3 mcg K_2/100G
* Soft cheeses—56.5 mcg K_2/100G
* Egg yolk (from eggs in the Netherlands)—32.1 mcg K_2/100G (approximately 6 yolks)
* Goose leg meat—31.0 mcg K_2/100G
* Curd cheeses—24.8 mcg K_2/100G
* Egg yolk (from eggs in the United States)—15.5 mcg K_2/100G (approximately 6 yolks)
* Butter—15.0 mcg K_2/100G
* Chicken liver—14.1 mcg K_2/100G

*A note about natto: We have read varying opinions about whether or not the type of K_2 provided by natto (known as MK-7) demonstrates the same properties as the K_2 found in grass-fed dairy and meat (MK-4). Including natto in your diet is certainly not a bad idea, because fermented foods are chock-full of health benefits. However, unless you are vegan, you may want to consider adding some animal-based sources and/or supplementing with high-vitamin butter oil.

Notice that butter is lower on this list, and 100 g of butter is about 7 tablespoons, providing only 15 mcg of K_2. To get 100 mcg of K_2 from butter alone, according to this list, you would need nearly six sticks of butter per day. Now, we eat A LOT of butter, but six sticks daily is too much, even for us. What we can't tell from this report is whether or not this butter was from grass-fed cows, which would make all the difference because conventional butter doesn't contain much vitamin K_2 at all.

You can also see that the egg yolk for the Netherlands contained DOUBLE the vitamin K_2 compared to the egg from the United States. Hmm. Perhaps that U.S. egg was from a conventional source and the Dutch egg from a pastured source?

Some say that fish eggs are also quite high in K_2. Certain cheeses such as Gouda do not need to be made from grass-fed milk because the culturing process produces vitamin K_2 in the finished cheese, but for nearly every other K_2-rich food, the pasture-raised component is essential.

HIGH-VITAMIN BUTTER OIL FOR VITAMIN K2

High-vitamin butter oil (HVBO) is a concentrated supplement made by centrifuging the oil of grass-fed butter to concentrate the vitamin density. In his book *Nutrition and Physical Degeneration*, Weston Price discussed the use of HVBO from fall and spring cows on pasture to maximize the health benefits of fermented cod liver oil (FCLO)—essentially, the fat-soluble vitamins A and D from the FCLO seem to work synergistically with vitamin K_2 (which Price referred to as "Activator X") from HVBO.

Because HVBO is technically classified as a food, not a supplement, the precise content of vitamin K_2 is not included on the label. It has been suggested, however, that the HVBO is estimated at eight times more potent than regular butter, putting HBVO near the top of our list above. HVBO is also lactose-free and very low in casein—safe for most individuals with sensitivity to dairy.

If you decide to supplement with HVBO, here are some tips on dosage: According to Ramiel Nagel, author of *Cure Tooth Decay*, for severe cavities or severe tooth pain or infection, you want ¾ teaspoon of fermented cod liver oil and ¾ teaspoon of butter oil daily. This is equivalent to 10 capsules of the FCLO/HVBO blend or 7 capsules of each individually. For maintenance dosages, use about half the amounts listed for adults.

It's likely that the similar dosage recommendations would be ideal for treatment or prevention of other disease or imbalances as well. While pregnancy is certainly not a disease, it is quite demanding on the body, so women who are trying to conceive, are pregnant, or are nursing should aim for the higher dosage range. At the time of this writing, there is no known toxicity if vitamin K_2 is taken in large dosages.

PROBIOTICS

You've heard about acidophilus in yogurt being good for you, right? You may even take a probiotic supplement or eat probiotic-rich foods for health benefits. But did you know there are more than four hundred strains of beneficial bacteria that all play different roles in the body? Good gut flora plays an essential role in reduced inflammation and disease prevention. Because supporting fertility is best done with a whole-person approach, the state of the gut flora is, in effect, a biomarker for the overall health of a woman's body.

In the past, humans ate food that came more directly from the earth—not transported across continents, not sprayed with bug and weed repellents, and not genetically engineered to resist decay. The former food was naturally rich in beneficial microflora, while the latter most certainly is not.

Even organic produce is often sprayed with bleach (which itself evaporates) to lengthen the shelf life at your overpriced health food store. So, to ensure your body's microflora thrives, it's essential to include probiotics in one form or another. For those with immune system issues, digestive issues, or gut flora imbalance, it's a good idea to eat probiotic-rich foods AND take a high-quality supplement.

PROBIOTIC FOODS

Yogurt is the probiotic food source most people recognize and consume, but there's a whole world of cultured and fermented foods available as well—including a variety of cultured dairy products, fermented fruits and vegetables, condiments, and drinks. While it may seem intimidating to create your own probiotic-rich foods, things such as home-made sauerkraut, home-brewed kombucha, and even cultured ketchup are both super easy to make and surprisingly affordable. For detailed recipes and instructions, check out our culture food recipes starting on page 85.

PROBIOTIC SUPPLEMENTS

Supplementation is the easiest and fastest way to ensure your body is populated with the adequate beneficial flora. When choosing a high-quality probiotic supplement, it's good to know that some must be refrigerated and others are shelf stable.

Some probiotics need to be refrigerated in order to keep the probiotics' cells more stable—these probiotics most closely resemble the beneficial bacteria from cultured foods. Shelf-stable probiotics generally do not need to be stored at cool temperatures. These are typically soil-based organisms that can survive more extreme conditions and temperatures. As a result, they also survive longer through the digestive tract. These types of supplements are particularly useful when traveling or for individuals who need more profound probiotic therapy.

Yet other probiotic supplements may have an enteric coating designed to delay release and ensure stomach acids don't destroy beneficial bacteria before they reach the gut. These types of pills can also be useful for traveling or for when the digestive tract needs deeper healing—such as extreme dysbiosis from antibiotic use.

Finally, pay attention to any additional ingredients in whichever supplements you choose. Avoid all supplements with highly processed ingredients and avoid probiotics that contain dairy if you're sensitive to dairy products.

The B-complex vitamins are a group of eight vitamins: B_1 (thiamine), B_2 (riboflavin), B_3 (niacin), B_5 (pantothenoic acid), B_7 (biotin), B_6 (pyridoxine), B_9 (folate), and B_{12} (cyanocobalamin). They are essential to a number of functions in the body, including the following:

* The breakdown of carbohydrates into glucose, which provides energy for the body
* The breakdown of fats and proteins, which aid in the function of the nervous system
* Muscle tone in the stomach and intestinal tract, including prevention of IBS
* Healthy functioning of many body parts, including eyes, mouth, skin, hair, and liver
* Detoxification from free radicals, which can lead to inflammation and disease

As per usual, we would much rather see you getting your Bs from food sources. Generally speaking, if you are following the dietary recommendations outlined in this book, you're getting plenty of B vitamins. Food sources rich in B vitamins include brewer's yeast, liver, properly prepared whole grains, nuts, milk, eggs, meats, fish, fruits, and leafy green vegetables. Take a look at our section on honoring sacred foods on page 57 for B vitamin powerhouses.

For vegetarians, those who are under high stress, or folks who don't eat a healthy diet, B vitamin supplementation may be necessary. Specific to women's health, B_6 is sometimes used as a remedy for PMS and morning sickness.

Vitamin B_{12} is not found in any plant foods, so deficiency shows up most commonly in strict vegetarians. B_{12} helps make all of the blood cells in our bodies and is required for the maintenance of nerve sheaths, and plays a role in the synthesis and repair of DNA. In order to assimilate B_{12}, it has to bind to a protein made in the stomach called intrinsic factor. Strict vegetarians and people who fail to produce intrinsic factor may require shots of vitamin B_{12}. Others should have no problem taking in abundant amounts through healthy animal sources.

Vitamin B_9 is commonly known as folic acid. Folic acid is actually the synthetic version of folate, and it works in concert with B_{12} in DNA synthesis, vital for the health of all the body's cells. Folic acid has to be converted to folate for your body to use it, so you're better off getting it from food sources if possible.

Your body needs more folate during pregnancy, and supplementation guidelines are more than double that of nonpregnant people. Folate requirements can be met by eating a real food diet including organ meats, but it is important to take special care that you are getting enough, as deficiency can lead to serious issues including spina bifida in the fetus. If you are not able to meet the minimum recommended dosage of folate (400 mcg) through food sources, it makes sense to consider a high-quality supplement. At extremely high dosages, synthetic folic acid may be toxic.

✳ THE MTHFR GENE ✳

In 2003, scientists completed a study that mapped the genes of humans, called the Human Genome Project. They discovered that a particular gene, called methylenetetrahydrofolate reductase (MTHFR), was defective in many people. The MTHFR gene is necessary for converting folate into an enzyme that is crucial to detoxifying your cells—a process called methylation. When the conversion doesn't happen properly, lots of health problems can ensue including recurrent miscarriage, spina bifida, early onset of heart disease, depression, Parkinson's disease, IBS, cancer, migraines, and many more.

While we can't do anything to change a defective gene, people with the MTHFR mutation can take a methylated form of folic acid and vitamin B_{12}, which helps with the conversion process it can't do on its own.

Lypo-Spheric glutathione is another important supplement to consider if you have this mutation, as the MTHFR gene plays a big role in making glutathione in the body, which is vital for your immune system and for lowering inflammation. The MTHFR mutation can be easily checked in by a simple blood test, and we think it's a good idea, especially if you've had more than one miscarriage. This is one instance where supplementation may be more important than relying on food alone.

MINERALS

Minerals are chemical compounds used by the body for almost every function, including building bones, making hormones, regulating your heartbeat, and keeping your cells hydrated through their role as electrolytes. While minerals should be easy to get through a balanced, real food diet, it's not always so easy these days. Minerals should occur abundantly in soil, but the introduction of chemical fertilizers and pesticides into our agricultural system has left much farmland devoid of minerals. This is yet another reason to purchase and consume organic, biodynamic food, because these sustainable farming practices don't deplete the land, and in the best cases, actually *improve* soil quality.

Minerals are found in food throughout the food chain, so a balanced diet of well-sourced real food should have you covered. To bolster your mineral consumption, be sure to also include plenty of mineral-rich salts including Celtic sea salt or Himalayan pink salt. Seaweeds and ocean seafood are all rich in minerals, too.

There are two kinds of minerals: macrominerals and trace minerals. As the name suggests, macrominerals are required by the body in larger amounts than their trace counterparts. Macrominerals include calcium, phosphorus, magnesium, sodium potassium, chloride, and sulfur. Trace minerals include iron, iodine, copper, zinc, cobalt selenium, fluoride, and manganese. Your mineral levels can be checked via a blood test. If your values come back low despite your nutrient-dense diet, we think it's best to supplement with only the one(s) that are low.

ANTIOXIDANTS

When we mention antioxidants, you may think of taking vitamin C to prevent a cold. Using this example, in Chinese medicine, we say that when your body is fighting an infection, Wind invades from the Exterior—allowing a pathogen (Heat, Cold, or Damp) to enter your body and take up residence between the skin and the muscles creating chills, fever, body aches, sore throat, etc.—the beginnings of a cold or flu.

While the imagery of weather patterns may seem too poetic to accurately define medical illness, Wind invasion is actually quite parallel to what actually happens when free radicals invade healthy cells, leaving the body more vulnerable to inflammation from allergens and infection from viruses and other pathogens.

Free radicals are uncharged molecules that have an unpaired electron and are consequently typically highly reactive and short-lived. To a certain extent, free radicals are unavoidable. They occur as a normal part of metabolism, and some are actually used as defense mechanisms by our immune system, but environment and lifestyle also introduce extra free radicals around every corner via car exhaust, pesticides, preservatives, and processed foods. Free radicals also multiply from poor lifestyle choices such as unmanaged stress or lack of sleep. These free radicals are the ones creating detrimental cell damage.

Antioxidants are like the bouncers that escort the riffraff out of a nightclub. Antioxidants do not directly act against viruses, bacteria, allergens, and other toxins but greatly reduce cell damage by neutralizing free radicals. When cells are not being damaged by free radicals, the body has more fortitude to defend against illness. Specifically regarding fertility, high levels of antioxidants can help protect egg and sperm quality.

ANTIOXIDANTS IN FOOD

It's best to get antioxidants from food, including seasonal fruits and vegetables, raw milk, and other "living" foods such as raw oysters and raw eggs from pasture-raised hens.

Many common foods, especially fruits, vegetables, spices, and oils, are rich sources of antioxidants (vitamins C and E, carotenoids, polyphenols, etc.), each having their own special way of functioning. The best way to make sure your body has the antioxidant support it needs is to consume a variety of antioxidant-rich food and—when necessary—antioxidant supplements.

A trip to the supplement section of your health food store in search of antioxidants may make you dizzy with choices. Below we will present three notable antioxidants, but it's worth remembering that these are only a few of the options available to you.

VITAMIN C

Vitamin C is an antioxidant powerhouse. Nearly anyone you ask will say a glass of orange juice is a great common cold remedy, and we even see gas stations selling individual packets of fizzy vitamin C. That said, all vitamin C is not equally beneficial to the body, and some may, in fact, be detrimental when taken routinely. In a bind, a few powdered vitamin C packets are not going to kill you, but we wouldn't suggest downing these on a daily basis.

When taking synthetic vitamin C for acute immune support (like to fend off a cold), you will often need a high dose for efficacy—2 to 4 grams for adults, spread throughout the day. Better yet, opt for food-based sources of vitamin C every day, including whatever fresh seasonal fruit your local farmer is growing at this time of year. When you use real food to get your nutrients, you not only get the nutrient itself, but also lots of cofactors (such as bioflavonoids) that make the nutrients more effective.

When you're deep in cold and flu season, around sick people (especially kids), or just starting to feel under the weather, take an extra boost of vitamin C using a natural supplement such as acerola or pure elderberry syrup.

GLUTATHIONE

Glutathione is a simple molecule that is produced all the time in your body. It's a combination of three amino acids—cysteine, glycine, and glutamine. Glutathione has been called the mother of all antioxidants—and for good reason. It contains unique sulfur compounds, which make them sticky (and stinky). The sticky quality of glutathione means that free radicals, mercury, and other heavy metals adhere to it, allowing these and other toxins to pass out of the body via bile and stool.

Aside from detoxification, glutathione is also crucial for energy production and proper functioning of the immune system—assisting other antioxidants in their jobs.

Normally, your body produces its own glutathione that it can recycle and reuse. Unfortunately, when the toxic load becomes too great (from poor diet, stress, trauma, pollution, aging, infections, radiation, etc.), your glutathione becomes depleted, leaving you vulnerable to cell damage from free radicals, infection, and abnormal cell growth. Without the protective function of glutathione, your liver can get overloaded, making it unable to do its job of detoxification.

Some people are better than others at detoxifying, often due to GSTM1, a gene essential to the process of creating and recycling glutathione in the body. Those with a MTHFR gene mutation will need supplementation since that gene plays a big role in glutathione production. That said, your ability to produce and maintain glutathione is essential to recovering from and preventing disease and maintaining optimal health and performance.

COQ$_{10}$

CoQ$_{10}$ (a.k.a. ubiquinone) assists mitochondrial function, which is the energy-producing center of each cell. Preliminary studies show that CoQ$_{10}$ can specifically improve sperm motility and count in men and may increase follicle count and pregnancy rates in females.

A typical dose of CoQ_{10} is 300 mg/day, but smaller, more frequent doses may help to maintain more stable blood levels, so some health practitioners recommend taking three doses per day of 100 mg each for more uniform energy production.

AMINO ACID THERAPY

Do you suffer from emotional imbalances or cravings for sugar, caffeine, or other substances? If so, it may be a bit overwhelming to ditch junk food or manage your stress to optimize fertility. Easier said than done, right? Luckily, there's something that may help.

Dr. Julia Ross, a researcher, clinician, and author of *The Mood Cure* and *The Diet Cure* has made some very interesting discoveries about our brain chemistry. She's found that many modern-day folks are living with neurotransmitter deficiencies leading to excessive cravings and mood imbalances.

Neurotransmitters conduct signals through the brain and nervous system and throughout the body. They are made from amino acids, which are also the building blocks of protein. Neurotransmitter deficiency can happen because you eat a poor diet lacking in enough protein to supply the right balance of amino acids. You can also become deficient if you don't get enough sleep or you have been under a lot of stress (either acute or chronic) from the loss of a loved one, financial strain, or say, fertility challenges. Whatever the reason, you undernourish and overtax your body to the point where you are severely deficient in one or more neurotransmitters, leading to cravings and emotional imbalance.

According to Dr. Ross, in two-thirds of individuals suffering from this type of imbalance, the deficiency is so profound that simply eating a really great diet will not be enough to correct the deficiency.

THE AMINO ACID SOLUTION

Instead of taking medication, which can further drive neurotransmitter deficiencies, you can supplement with the amino acid precursors our bodies need to correct the imbalance. If you're eating a nutrient-rich diet, that period of supplementation will likely have to last for a few months—or just long enough to resolve the deficiency. Once resolved, your diet can supply all you need unless stress and fatigue get the better of you again.

DETERMINING A NEUROTRANSMITTER DEFICIENCY

Ross presents four different types of neurotransmitter deficiencies: serotonin, catecholamine, GABA, and endorphin. She also addresses hypoglycemia. To be sure of your specific deficiencies and determine your correct dosage of amino acid therapy, we recommend reading one or both of Julia Ross's books and/or working with a qualified health practitioner familiar with amino acid therapy.

Let's look at each type of neurotransmitter deficiency, its related symptoms and craving, and the amino acid that can correct the imbalance.

NEUROTRANSMITTER DEFICIENCIES & AMINO ACID RECOMMENDATIONS

Neurotransmitter Deficiency	Common Symptoms	Common Substances Used	Amino Acid Therapy	Therapeutic Goal
Serotonin	• Afternoon or evening cravings for specific food/substances • Negativity, depression, worry, anxiety, low self-esteem, obsessive thoughts or behaviors, controlling, perfectionism, or suicidal thoughts • Winter blues, dislikes hot weather • Irritability, rage (PMS), or panic attacks/phobias • TMJ (jaw pain) or other chronic pain, such as fibromyalgia • Night owl, insomnia, or disturbed sleep	• Sweets and starch Tobacco Chocolate Ecstasy Marijuana Alcohol Prozac Zoloft Paxil Effexor Celexa	5-HTP L-tryptophan Melatonin for sleep at bedtime	• Positive outlook • Emotional stability • Self-confidence • Emotional and mental flexibility • Sense of humor
Catecholamine	• Crave stimulation from sugar, chocolate, caffeine, cocaine, or meth • Depression, apathy • Lack of energy, drive, focus, and/or concentration; ADHD; or hyperactivity	• Sweets and starch • Tobacco • Chocolate • Aspartame • Marijuana • Caffeine • Cocaine • Diet pills • Wellbutrin • Ritalin • Adderall	L-tyrosine	• Alertness • Energy • Mental focus • Drive • Enthusiasm
GABA	• Crave carbs, alcohol, or drugs for relaxation • Stressed and burned out, unable to relax/loosen up • Stiff or tense muscles • Often feel easily overwhelmed	• Tobacco • Alcohol • Marijuana • Valium • Ativan • Neurontin • Klonopin	GABA	• Calmness • Relaxation • Stress tolerance
Endorphin	• Crave comfort, reward, or numbing treats • "Love" certain foods, behaviors, drugs, or alcohol • Sensitive to emotional or physical pain, cries (tear up) easily	• Sweets and starch • Tobacco • Alcohol • Marijuana • Chocolate • Caffeine • Vicodin • Heroin	DL or D-Phenylalanine	Psychosocial and physical pain relief and tolerance Pleasure, reward, and loving feelings

∼ Choosing a *Real* Prenatal Vitamin ∽

We've made our case for why food can and should be adequate nutrition. If you still want extra insurance, it's worthwhile to choose a prenatal vitamin that your body can actually digest and utilize.

Most prenatal vitamins contain the synthetic form of many key nutrients. For example, folic acid sits in for folate, and carotenoids are offered in place of vitamin A. Synthetic forms and precursors do not always act the same as the required nutrient, so the body has to work harder to compensate.

Research has shown that the ability to absorb usable nutrients from prenatal multivitamins is often inadequate. For example, a 1997 report published in the *Journal of the American Pharmacists Association*, called "Failure of Prescription Prenatal Vitamin Products to Meet USP Standards for Folic Acid Dissolution," states that folic acid content was below industry standards in more than two-thirds of those tested. Additionally, contaminants such as lead (a leading cause of developmental issues in children) have been found in commercial prenatals.

Many women have health insurance coverage for prenatal vitamins that are prescribed by their doctor, and for that reason, decide to take them instead of a food-based alternative. While we understand it's nice to pinch pennies, we also think that (if at all possible) this is not the place to cut corners. Investing in high-quality supplements dramatically increases their bioavailability and cuts down on the risk of contaminants, which are often found in large commercial brands. While prescription brands might be slightly higher quality than their big-box store competitors, they are still synthetic and should be avoided if possible.

The best way to protect oneself from contaminants and low nutrient absorption is to seek out a prenatal vitamin that is from whole food sources. These can often be acquired through your local health food store, online, or through a qualified holistic practitioner.

Part 3

Dealing with Obstacles—
Conventional and Holistic Solutions for Common Infertility Issues

In this section, we will review many of the common fertility obstacles that arise, and with each one, we will outline the Western and Chinese medicine perspectives, plus the common medical treatments that are used. We've also included some case studies of real patients (with fictional names) to demonstrate how fertility can be cultivated in the presence of challenges.

....

Chapter 1

Advanced Maternal Age— Am I Too Old to Have a Baby?

THESE DAYS, MANY WOMEN EARN GRADUATE DEGREES, pursue careers, or simply wait for the right partner before settling down to get married and/or have families. While we're all for women's rights, there is one unfortunate hitch in this plan: **biology**.

Realistically, many women in their 40s will have a heck of a time getting pregnant because that's how most of us are genetically programmed. Painful as it might be, it's helpful to consider that women who conceive naturally later in life are the exception to the rule—*outliers*, if you will. If you are struggling with fertility in your late 30s or 40s, you don't have a disease. Your body is going through the normal functions associated with your age. Despite the inevitable aging timeline, there are ways via both science and nature to improve your pregnancy odds.

～ What the West Says ～
....

The media shows us attractive women in their late 40s happily pushing infant twins in a stroller on the way to the park and presents research indicating that older women will have smarter and healthier babies. What tabloids don't reveal, however, is how many cycles of IVF failed before a successful pregnancy occurred, how much medication the mother needed to inject and ingest, how many tens of thousands of dollars had been spent, and if these babies were born via donor egg, donor sperm, and/or a gestational carrier to host the pregnancy.

Reproductive medicine can be a miracle of science, but it is an extremely expensive (and often emotionally draining) miracle, yielding lower and lower margins of success with each passing year of age.

That said, we believe that knowledge is power. We recommend that all women over the age of 40 who have been trying for more than three months seek a Western workup with a reproductive endocrinologist to rule out potential obstacles to conception—whether hormonal or structural. It is better to do this at the outset, rather than allowing precious time to go by. Some conditions (such as fibroid removal) can take several months in the healing process, so determining and treating any issues detracting from your fertility right away may make a big difference in your success.

～ Genetics and Epigenetics: Why Some "Older" Women Can Conceive and Others Cannot ～

How long we are able to procreate is different for every person. Just because your best friend's sister-in-law's cousin got pregnant at 48 doesn't mean we all can. Trying to change your genetics around your fertility is as futile as trying to have blue eyes just because someone else does.

What we can influence, however, is epigenetics. Epigenetics is defined as the way our genes express themselves. This emerging field is providing more and more evidence that the things we do, like how we eat, think, and feel, can actually influence the way our genetic predispositions play out. For example, just because you have a family history of breast cancer doesn't mean you are doomed to develop this disease yourself. Likewise, while your waning fertility may be a natural part of your genetic programming, you can slow this process a bit and optimize pregnancy outcomes by making smart choices in how you choose to live your life.

Changing your diet, lifestyle habits, self-care routines, and stress levels can go a long way toward turning back the biological clock. Regardless of whether or not you end up having a biological child, these methods will only bring you better health and vitality, which is what you need to be a parent, biological or otherwise.

～ What the East Says ～

While Western medicine has very little to offer in terms of turning back your biological clock, Chinese medicine can help to breathe hope and inspiration into the space where your odds seem to decline with each passing month.

Chinese medical texts say that pregnancy should be possible from the onset of our first period (menarche) through the very last (menopause). With that in mind, let's examine how Chinese medicine can help to optimize fertility through influencing epigenetics well into your later reproductive years.

Depending on a woman's reproductive profile, Chinese medicine can often dramatically slow down and sometimes even reverse ovarian decline. We have personally assisted many patients with "rebooting" their ovaries, which can increase follicle count, improve responses to fertility drugs, and result in more pregnancies (natural or assisted) and fewer miscarriages.

Having a healthy, regular menstrual cycle is the cornerstone of improving fertility health, and Chinese medicine shines when it comes to this. Using herbs and acupuncture to regulate and support the cycle, women may find themselves ovulating and menstruating more regularly, experiencing less pain and clotting, feeling less PMS, having better cervical fluid at ovulation, and experiencing an improved libido.

Beyond the mere functionality of your reproductive organs and hormones, Chinese medicine can help you to cultivate fertility in your entire being, so that you can approach your baby-making journey from a place of feeling already fulfilled by your life, rather than trying to fill an empty space in your heart with a baby.

IT'S A JING THING

As you now know, Jing is the sacred stuff imparted to us through our genes at the time we are conceived. It's finite, and it declines as we age. Our own genetic material (eggs and sperm) is made from Jing, which explains why so many are chromosomally abnormal in older women—it's a normal response to aging.

Chinese medicine works hard to support the Jing you've still got, by offering powerful herbs, effective acupuncture, and meaningful lifestyle and dietary recommendations. If you do your part (showing up, taking your herbs, and making any suggested lifestyle changes), you will likely see some tangible improvements in both your reproductive and overall health.

Since the Kidneys house the Jing, which rules reproductive health and genetics, Chinese medicine treatments for advanced maternal age will virtually always incorporate strategies that support the Kidney system.

✳ HANNAH'S STORY ✳

Hannah, 39, was trying to conceive and suffering from moderate anxiety, depression, and headaches. She often had very long cycles with no sign of ovulation on her predictor sticks, an indication of oligo-ovulation ("ovulating some of the time"). I sent her for the standard testing and while her FSH* was normal, her progesterone was slightly low and her AMH* was 0.4, indicating a very low ovarian reserve. Her reproductive endocrinologist advised her that her best option was to immediately pursue IVF. Because Hannah and her husband couldn't afford this treatment, she decided to decline Western medical options and stick with acupuncture, Chinese herbs, diet, and lifestyle adjustments.

We focused heavily on Jing foods and stress management for Hannah. She came weekly for acupuncture and took herbs to encourage ovulation. Within a few months, she began ovulating nearly every cycle.

Toward the second half of the year, Hannah got pregnant three times and experienced very early miscarriages, often referred to as "biochemical pregnancies." The month of her 40th birthday, she called to tell me she was pregnant again. She and her husband recently welcomed a healthy little girl.
See Understanding the Basic Fertility Workup on page 189 for a more detailed explanation of these terms.

✳ ANNIE'S STORY ✳

Annie, 43, was just beginning her first IVF cycle. Already the mother of a five-year-old son, she was determined to have another child as quickly as possible. Because her IVF cycle had already begun, it was too late to influence her constitution or egg count/quality. She had regular acupuncture sessions throughout the cycle and during the two-week waiting period between her embryo transfer and pregnancy test. Unfortunately, she did not achieve pregnancy.

She decided to wait a few months before trying IVF again. She continued receiving weekly acupuncture, took Chinese herbs, and improved her diet by eating more healthy fats and organic food, sticking to regular mealtimes, and increasing her calories overall. She also worked on managing her stress levels.

Her next IVF cycle was much better, with a higher follicle count at the start, and overall excellent progress. A positive pregnancy test led to the discovery of two heartbeats! Though her pregnancy was challenging, she delivered two healthy baby girls.

Chapter 2

Miscarriage

WHETHER OR NOT GETTING PREGNANT COMES EASILY TO YOU, not every pregnancy "sticks." Pregnancy loss can be an agonizing experience. For women undergoing fertility treatments, the devastation that comes with miscarriage is compounded—all the visits to the doctor, untold dollars spent, and life put on hold—simply adding insult to an already significant loss.

∼ What the West Says ∼

Miscarriage, clinically referred to as spontaneous abortion, and defined as the spontaneous loss of pregnancy before the 20th week, is much more common than most people realize. According to the American Pregnancy Association, 10 to 25 percent of known pregnancies end in miscarriage, but many more than that occur because they happen before a woman even realizes she is pregnant. In fact, up to 75 percent of all pregnancy losses are what are called "chemical pregnancies," where the miscarriage occurs shortly after implantation and the period arrives just a few days late.

Often we don't find out exactly what caused a miscarriage, though statistically we do know that most pregnancies end because the fetus isn't growing properly, usually caused by chromosomal abnormalities.

Women sometimes take miscarriage very personally, often blaming themselves and creating a belief system that their bodies have failed them. The truth is, this is rarely the case. While the experience of loss can bring sadness, miscarriage is a common reality for women of childbearing age.

∼ What *Won't* Cause Miscarriage ∼

When pregnancies end, women will often try and think back over *everything* they have done since the day they conceived, in an effort to pinpoint a reason for their loss. Not only is this practice quite unproductive, it's also myth driven. Let's take a look at what *doesn't* cause miscarriage, so you can give yourself a break:

* **EXERCISE**—Getting your heart rate up won't make you lose your baby. That said, pregnancy is not a time to train for a marathon or start a new rigorous fitness routine, unless you were doing those things before you conceived.
* **SEX**—Sometimes sexual intercourse can lead to a bit of cramping, but it typically passes pretty quickly and will not dislodge a healthy pregnancy. That said, if your doctor recommends that you abstain for a period of time, please heed his or her advice.
* **WORK**—While you may be looking for a reason to stay home and watch streaming TV shows, doing your regular job won't cause you to lose your baby. You should, of course, avoid exposure to toxic chemicals and radiation.
* **STRESS**—While too much stress in and of itself is not healthy or ideal in pregnancy, it's not likely to be the cause of miscarriage on its own. If stress alone induced miscarriages, we'd have a lot fewer people on the planet.

∼ Common Causes of Miscarriage ∽

There are some general risk factors that increase a woman's potential for miscarriage including age, history of miscarriages (more than two), being overweight or underweight, smoking, alcohol and drug use, and invasive prenatal tests to check for chromosomal issues—including CVS and amniocentesis. Issues with the sperm and egg quality and health issues with the prospective mother can also lead to miscarriage.

CHROMOSOMAL ABNORMALITIES

Chromosomal abnormalities are the most common cause of miscarriage. At the time of conception, the egg and sperm have to meet, divide, and grow. This process is immensely complex, and errors frequently happen along the way resulting in conditions such as Down syndrome. Inherited genetic abnormalities—such as cystic fibrosis—are when one or both parents are the carriers of a disease.

Some of the most common examples of miscarriage due to chromosomal abnormalities include the following:

* **BLIGHTED OVUM**—This happens when fertilization and implantation take place, but the embryo doesn't grow. On ultrasound, it looks like an empty sac.
* **INTRAUTERINE FETAL DEMISE**—This occurs when a pregnancy has been established, but the fetus stops growing before any signs of miscarriage. In this case, and depending on how far along she is, a woman may choose to undergo a D&C or allow her body to spontaneously miscarry.

HEALTH ISSUES IN THE MOM-TO-BE

Expectant moms with certain health issues may be at greater risk for miscarriage. If you have been diagnosed with any one of the following, it is important to be under the care of a qualified medical doctor and possibly a fertility specialist *before* you become pregnant, so you can be carefully monitored to avoid problems:

* **UNCONTROLLED DIABETES:** It is crucial to make sure you are eating properly and that your medications are properly dosed to avoid complications in your pregnancy.
* **INFECTIONS:** Certain infections can cause an increase in miscarriage risk including bacterial vaginosis, chlamydia, rubella, toxoplasmosis, and certain foodborne illnesses, such as listeria.
* **LUTEAL PHASE DEFECT:** After ovulation, the outer shell of the follicle, called the corpus luteum, stays in the ovary and produces the hormone progesterone. Progesterone is vital to pregnancy, and a defective corpus luteum that doesn't make enough, or peters out too soon, can cause an otherwise healthy pregnancy to end.
* **UTERINE AND CERVICAL ISSUES:** Structural issues in the uterus, such as septum, bicornuate shape, or fibroids pushing into the cavity, can all impact the ability to hold a pregnancy. A weak cervix, often the result of surgical procedures, can also make it difficult to maintain a pregnancy to term.
* **AUTOIMMUNE DISEASE:** Conditions such as lupus, rheumatoid arthritis, and other diseases where the immune system becomes overactive and attacks itself are associated with an increased rate of miscarriage.
* **THYROID DISEASE:** Thyroid issues can cause a myriad of fertility-related problems including miscarriage. See page 174 for more about thyroid conditions and fertility.

~ Western Treatment for Recurrent Miscarriages ~

Western medicine has a small bag of tricks when it comes to preventing miscarriage. The primary treatments include the following:

* Progesterone supplementation for those who are low
* Aspirin to thin the blood and help with implantation/blood clotting problems
* Heparin for known clotting disorders
* Steroids to suppress the immune system for people with overactive immune responses that might be attacking the developing embryo/fetus

∽ **What the East Says** ∾

Chinese medicine can be an extremely useful tool in preventing miscarriage, unless the fetus is not chromosomally normal. In the case of chromosomal abnormalities, nature will usually stop the pregnancy on its own, and Chinese medicine can support the mother's physical and emotional recovery. If medical intervention is required (such as a D&C), Chinese medicine can assist with healing and preparing the body for getting pregnant again.

With regard to recurrent miscarriage, Chinese herbs have proven to be quite effective when it comes to treatment, especially when the loss is caused by an overactive immune system or autoimmune disease.

Chinese medicine looks at an individual's diagnosis to determine how to bring the body into balance in order to protect the pregnancy or prevent future pregnancy loss. Aside from the waning of Jing that comes with age, miscarriage may be caused by Kidney deficiency, Qi deficiency, heat in the Blood, or Blood stagnation. Refer to the section on Chinese medicine and fertility on page 45 to learn more about each of these diagnoses.

✳ JANE'S STORY ✳

Jane, a 37-year-old mother of one, came in after having a recent miscarriage. Though she had conceived her first child easily, getting pregnant a second time had proved more difficult. Finally, she became pregnant after six months of trying, only to discover that her fetus no longer had a heartbeat at eight weeks. A D&C was performed, and two cycles had passed before she came to see me. She was clearly run down and stressed from the obligations of taking care of a young toddler, suffering from insufficient sleep, and paying little attention to her diet. Her diagnosis was Spleen Qi and Liver Blood deficiency. Through a combination of acupuncture, Chinese herbs to build her Blood and Qi, and a focus on sufficient sleep and healthy food, Jane became pregnant within two more cycles. She gave birth to a healthy baby girl.

Chapter 3

Endometriosis, Fibroids, and Polyps

ENDOMETRIOSIS, FIBROIDS, AND POLYPS are all conditions where abnormal growth of tissue occurs either inside or outside of the uterus. While all three are diagnosed as different conditions in Western medicine, from a Chinese medicine perspective, the causes and treatments have many commonalities.

∼ Endometriosis ∼

Endometriosis is a condition where the tissue that normally grows inside the uterus, called the endometrium, implants itself and grows outside of the uterus. When a woman starts her period, the irregular tissue bleeds into the pelvic cavity, causing pain, inflammation, and scarring. It is estimated that endometriosis affects 20 to 40 percent of women with infertility.

WHAT THE WEST SAYS

While there is no absolute certainty as to how or why endometriosis occurs, some common theories include the following:

* A backflow of menstruation through the fallopian tubes, leading to implantation of endometrial tissue in the peritoneal cavity. This could be caused by a tight cervical opening to the vagina, which in turn makes it difficult for menstrual flow to get out.
* Endometrial tissue growing in the wrong place when the baby was developing in utero. This theory speaks to the rare (but not unheard of) placement of endometrial lesions outside of the peritoneal cavity (in the chest or nasal cavity, for example).
* Genetic predisposition

Endometriosis can only be diagnosed through laparoscopic surgery. Symptoms that might lead a physician to suspect endometriosis include pelvic pain, painful periods, severe cramping and spotting before menstruation, PMS, pain with sexual intercourse, infertility, and digestive complaints such as diarrhea, constipation, and painful defecation, especially during menstruation.

The frequency and severity of symptoms do not necessarily correspond with the number or severity of lesions. Women with minor endometriosis can suffer terribly, while others with implants that are severely impacting their fertility may be fairly asymptomatic.

HOW DOES ENDOMETRIOSIS CAUSE INFERTILITY?

* Irregular tissue formation can distort the shape and position of the fallopian tubes and/or ovaries.
* Mucus produced by the implants can fill the fallopian tubes, preventing the eggs from getting through.
* Endometrial cysts (a.k.a. endometriomas or chocolate cysts) can grow inside the ovaries, causing inflammation and damaging the ovarian cortex where eggs develop
* Inflammation leads to an increase in white blood cells (macrophages), which can also attack sperm and embryos.
* Endometriosis is associated with low progesterone levels and may contribute to implantation problems.

Endometriosis is very difficult to cure, and most Western medical treatment is aimed at reducing the severity of symptoms, including pain and infertility. Laparoscopic surgery is the primary tool used by medical doctors to "clean up" the peritoneal cavity of lesions, cysts, and scar tissue.

Hormone treatments are also common. By suppressing a woman's menstrual cycle with medications such as the birth control pill, or stronger suppressors such as Lupron, less endometrial tissue will grow, both inside and outside the uterus. For women trying to conceive, suppressive hormone treatment is not an option because it suppresses ovulation and normal reproductive function.

The symptoms of endometriosis have been recognized by Chinese medicine for millennia, although the disease itself was never formally named. When viewed through the lens of Chinese medicine, Kidney Jing deficiency with Blood stagnation is generally the underlying cause of endometriosis. Other causes are possible, including the following:

* **IMPEDED QI FLOW** (Liver Qi stagnation, which is caused by emotional upset and leads to Blood stagnation)
* **INTERNAL COLD CONDITIONS** (think congealed blood that can't move), leading to stagnation and pain (this could be caused by too much exposure to cold at a young age)
* **SPLEEN DEFICIENCY**, which will impact digestion and the body's production of new blood

Similar to the Western viewpoint, Blood stasis leads to pathological heat symptoms (inflammation), which in turn triggers an immune response intended to protect the body from this pathological fluid (blood lesions in an inappropriate place in the body). Unfortunately, this "attack" by the immune system ends up doing more harm than good, leading to the symptoms described above.

According to studies compiled by the Cochrane Database, Chinese herbal formulas have shown to be equally or more effective than Western medical treatments in treating endometriosis and associated inflammation. Chinese medicine has also been proven to significantly reduce pain and has the added effect of helping to balance hormones and improve overall reproductive health. Western medical treatments such as Lupron or Danazol appear to be slightly less beneficial than herbs, and they don't treat the underlying cause or do much to balance the reproductive system.

Acupuncture is extremely effective in the treatment of pain associated with endometriosis. It modulates the brain's pain response through the release of internal pain reducers called opioids and reduces stress levels, which can subdue the intensity of pain. Acupuncture also plays a role in enhancing the positive effects of herbs and good diet. For example, needling points that correspond with the endocrine system will support and enhance herbs and foods intended to regulate the same system.

≈ Fibroids and Polyps ≈
....

Fibroids are noncancerous growths that form in the muscle layer of the uterus, often during peak years for baby-making. Fibroids either push toward the outside of the uterus (subserosal), hang out in the muscle layer itself (intramural), or push into the uterine cavity (submucosal). Some fibroids are pedunculated, which means it hangs from

✳ TREATING ENDOMETRIOSIS THROUGH DIET AND LIFESTYLE ✳

As with many of the conditions we are discussing in this book, there is an association between endometriosis and prolonged exposure to stress. According to a 2006 study published in the *Brazilian Journal of Medical and Biological Research*, women with endometriosis tend to have an increase in both cortisol and prolactin levels (both associated with stress), which may explain why the condition is associated with decreased progesterone levels and infertility.

FOODS TO RESOLVE BLOOD STAGNATION: The focus for people with active endometriosis is to resolve Blood stagnation and clear heat, which is Chinese medicine-speak for reducing inflammation and calming the immune system. Whatever the initial reason for endometriosis, the end result is an overactive immune system trying to manage the situation, which results in more inflammation.

If there was ever a condition that called for ditching junk food, this is it. Women with endometriosis tend to benefit significantly from cutting out inflammatory foods, such as refined sugar, wheat, pasteurized dairy products and caffeine. Because the lesions respond to hormonal stimulation, special care should be paid to avoiding xenoestrogens, including soy and excessive environmental exposure (such as plastic).

FOODS FOR DIGESTIVE HEALTH: Depending on your overall pattern, it is always important to consider gut health when there is any inflammatory condition, and this is no exception. Cultured, probiotic-rich foods are a crucial component to reducing the inflammatory cascade initiated by the presence of endometriosis. If you have a history of yeast infections, chronic colds, food allergies, or candida, consider a diet intended to heal leaky gut syndrome, such as the GAPS diet.

a stalk into the uterine cavity, or toward the outer layer. If you're guessing that the kind that pushes or hangs into the cavity is the most likely to affect fertility, you are correct. Submucosal fibroids can push into the uterus, which can get in the way of implantation, especially when they are on the top part, called the fundus, where implantation usually happens. In rare cases, fibroids can actually compete for fetal blood supply and cause miscarriage.

Common symptoms of fibroids include heavy periods, menstrual flow that lasts a week or more, backache or pain that shoots into the legs, pressure or pain in the pelvic region, frequent urination or frequent urges with difficulty urinating, and constipation or rectal pressure.

Uterine polyps are caused by an overgrowth of tissue attached to the uterine lining by a base or a stalk. Polyps are usually benign, but some can be precancerous and, rarely, cancerous. They can be smaller than a sesame seed or as big as a table tennis ball. An individual might have one polyp or many (we've seen people with hundreds). Polyps are most common in perimenopausal and menopausal women, though it's not unheard of for younger women to get them, too. In terms of fertility, the presence of a polyp can sometimes disrupt implantation.

Often, polyps go undetected. Signs you might have them include very heavy menstrual bleeding, periods that are irregular in frequency and duration, bleeding between periods, or infertility.

Like endometriosis, fibroids are related to Blood stagnation in Chinese medicine. Polyps, on the other hand, tend to be caused by insufficient Qi allowing the outpouching of the uterine wall. Despite this slightly different etiology, the Western treatment is usually the same—surgery. The bottom line with both of these conditions comes down to a cost/benefit analysis in terms of how quickly you desire to become pregnant. For women of advanced maternal age, or other serious fertility challenges, attempting to resolve fibroids or polyps (that might be affecting implantation) through acupuncture, herbs, and diet alone might prove too lengthy a process.

Herbal treatments for these conditions can be very effective, but they can also take a long time to work. If you wanted a baby yesterday, you might decide that a surgical option makes the most sense for you. Herbs, acupuncture, and nutrition can aid tremendously in the healing process, helping to prepare your body to conceive.

Christie came in for acupuncture treatment at the age of 33 after battling endometriosis since puberty. She had undergone several laparoscopic surgeries, the most recent just one year earlier. Christie's life was quite stressful, as she had to wake up before dawn each day in order to get to her job, which was over an hour drive in heavy traffic. She suffered from chronic lack of sleep and ate a lot of processed convenience foods.

She suffered terribly from menstrual cramps, which began approximately one week prior to the start of her period. Her periods were heavy and very painful, often resulting in days of missed work and the use of pain medication.

After three months of acupuncture and herbal treatment, Christie's cramps had all but disappeared. She modified her lifestyle to ensure that she was getting enough sleep, even taking naps during her lunch hour. She also began eating more fresh food and cut most of the processed foods out of her diet. Still, she wasn't pregnant.

An HSG test revealed that the endometriosis had damaged her fallopian tubes, which were now filled with fluid. This condition, called hydrosalpynx, meant that her tubes needed to be removed if she hoped to conceive, because the fluid in her tubes was preventing the eggs from getting through. Even with IVF, the fluid could reflux into the uterus and possibly damage an implanting embryo. Without fallopian tubes, her only hopes for conception were via IVF.

After the surgery, Christie began an IVF cycle. Because of all of the damage to her ovaries from endometriosis, she had very few eggs. On the day of her embryo transfer, only one remained.

Two weeks later, she was pregnant . . . with identical twins—her one little embryo had divided! Today, they are healthy, thriving toddlers.

Chapter 4

Irregular or No Ovulation

IN ORDER TO GET PREGNANT, you need sperm, egg, and a uterus, so fertility challenges certainly arise when ovulation is irregular or not happening at all.

Some women do not ovulate regularly, often leading to a halt in menstrual periods, a condition called amenorrhea. In this section, we will discuss one cause: hypothalamic amenorrhea (HA), but amenorrhea can also be caused by hyperprolactinemia (high levels of prolactin), ovulatory disorders, including PCOS, and other, rare causes.

◌ **What the West Says** ◌

The hypothalamus sits at the base of your brain and effectively serves as the command center for just about all of your body's functions. It serves as the mediator between the nervous system and the endocrine system, by telling the pituitary (an almond-shaped gland behind the center of your forehead) which hormones to secrete. The hypothalamic-pituitary-ovarian axis (HPO axis) refers to the interactive relationship between the hypothalamus, pituitary, and the reproductive system.

Sometimes the hypothalamus doesn't function properly. There are several reasons why this can happen:

* Poor nutrition and severe calorie restriction, as often seen in women with eating disorders
* Sudden extreme weight loss
* Overexercise or extreme athleticism (i.e., young competitive gymnasts)
* Extreme stress, often prolonged
* Unknown (idiopathic) causes

Because the hypothalamus controls reproductive hormones, amenorrhea, anovulation, and infertility can arise when it doesn't function properly.

Hypothalamic amenorrhea (HA) ranges from poor function to complete ovarian shutdown and cessation of menstruation. HA differs from advanced maternal age or premature ovarian failure because in this case the *brain* is the reason for the diminished action, not the ovaries themselves.

For younger women, this can be good news. Because both Chinese and Western medicine can assist in getting the hypothalamus back online, once things are up and running there's a good chance that the eggs are still healthy enough to make a healthy baby. Depending on the severity, women with this condition may require hormone support throughout much of their pregnancy.

∼ Diagnosis of Hypothalamic Amenorrhea ∽

Lab work for patients with HA will often show very low FSH, estradiol, and LH levels. This is because in women with HA, the HPO-axis is not working properly and the end result is that the ovaries don't get the signal to ovulate via the hypothalamus and pituitary gland.

Another diagnostic tool is called a "progesterone challenge." If a woman isn't getting her period and is given progesterone, her period should start shortly after she stops taking it (the same way you get your period a day or two into the placebo pills in birth control packs). In the case of women with hypothalamic amenorrhea, progesterone alone won't induce a period because her lining is too thin to shed. Consequently, a woman with HA will need estrogen to build her lining followed by progesterone to make her period start.

∼ Medical Treatment of Hypothalamic Amenorrhea ∽

Lifestyle changes are the best treatment for hypothalamic amenorrhea. Learning to manage stress, seeking treatment for eating disorders, gaining sufficient weight, and reducing exercise to appropriate levels goes a long way in giving the hypothalamus a kick start.

Fertility drugs for promoting ovulation and menstruation are the most common form of treatment offered by Western medicine, and IVF is often recommended.

Women with this condition should seek regular medical care and work hard to maintain a healthy diet, as there is an increased risk of osteoporosis and heart disease associated with this condition.

∼ The Importance of Diet and Lifestyle for Hypothalamic Amenorrhea ∼

A woman with hypothalamic amenorrhea should first determine if her condition is due to insufficient food intake, and if so, she must take action to increase her calorie consumption because restricting food is simply incompatible with a healthy pregnancy. For women with a history of calorie restricting or other eating disorders, appropriate mental and emotional support should be sought, in addition to nutritional changes.

Once eating is restored to normal quantities and frequency, focusing on digestion is the next, most important step. Balancing intestinal bacteria with cultured foods, probiotic supplements, and digestive enzymes (if necessary) will help to restore the body's ability to assimilate nutrition, allowing it to heal. Consuming lots of bone broth is key to healing the digestive tract and improving nutrient assimilation, so soups and broths are perfect foods to focus on, especially at the beginning.

Once digestion is working well, the main focus should be on foods to nourish Jing and to build Qi and Blood. It is vital to eat enough healthy saturated fat, in order that the body has enough building blocks to make hormones.

While we hope that any imbalances that have arisen as a result of a dysfunctional hypothalamus can be corrected through natural means alone, this may not always be possible. Some women's reproductive systems have been shut down for so long that a jump start of hormone therapy is required to get things moving again. The need for this depends on age and how much time you're willing to dedicate to reversing your condition. In some cases, even after some hormonal supplementation, follicle counts remain very low due to having your ovaries in a resting state for too long. In this case, medications that stimulate the ovaries may be helpful, either in conjunction with IUI or IVF.

∼ What the East Says ∼

In terms of stimulating the hypothalamus, two acupuncture channels—the Ren Mai and the Du Mai—have the greatest influence. Part of the Eight Extraordinary Meridian system, these two channels form a closed loop called the Microcosmic Orbit, which can be superimposed right over the HPO axis, and thereby have direct impact on its function. By stimulating the HPO axis, hormone function will begin to restore, along with better Qi and Blood flow to the uterus.

Suppressed hypothalamic function can also cause the nervous system to be out of balance, generating anxiety, fear, and stress, even when the situation at hand doesn't warrant it. Acupuncture is also one of the best methods for addressing this imbalance.

Herbal medicine for hypothalamic amenorrhea focuses on the phasic treatments we have discussed in previous sections, with special attention paid to Jing herbs because the brain is governed by the Kidney system in Chinese medicine, which is made of Jing.

✳ KATIE'S STORY ✳

Katie came into my office at 34 years of age, after several years of amenorrhea. Her periods stopped coming soon after a serious car accident years earlier, and she was told by two different OB-GYNs that she was postmenopausal. This was devastating news to her, as she desperately wanted a child.

I sent her for a workup with a reproductive endocrinologist. Her labs showed very low FSH* and LH* levels, common to HA. Ultrasound confirmed that her ovaries were not producing any follicles, and her uterine lining was extremely thin. She also had a sluggish thyroid and was given medication to correct it.

The doctor felt that she needed to start having regular menstrual cycles in order to protect herself from uterine cancer and to get her ovaries working again. She was administered estrogen and progesterone, and after several months, began showing some ovarian activity, but not enough to pursue IVF (IUI was not an option for her because her husband had serious sperm issues).

For seven months, she took strong Chinese herbs focused on healing her metabolism, warming her uterus, and regulating her hormones. She came in for acupuncture every week without fail. She made a complete overhaul of her diet, introducing meat, butter, and many traditional foods that she had long avoided.

Finally the day came to begin IVF. Her follicle counts were still quite low, but she responded well to the medications and the cycle went off without a hitch. When the day came to transfer embryos, there was just one four-cell remaining. Nine months later, a beautiful baby boy arrived.

*See the section Understanding the Basic Fertility Workup (page 189) for a more detailed explanation of these terms.

Chapter 5
....

Polycystic Ovary
Syndrome (PCOS)

POLYCYSTIC OVARY SYNDROME (PCOS) is the most common hormonal disorder, inflicting as many as 1 in 10 women of childbearing age in the United States, and according to the Office on Women's Health, it is the largest known cause of female infertility.

≈ **What the West Says** ≈

PCOS is a syndrome that is diagnosed when an individual meets two out of three symptoms in the diagnosis criteria:
* Ovaries that are enlarged and appear to have many "cysts" around the outer edge (sometimes called a ring of pearls)
* Irregular ovulation or anovulation
* Hirsutism—a condition caused by increased androgens (male hormones) in the bloodstream, leading to male pattern hair growth (chin, chest, and abdomen), hair loss/thinning (head), and acne

    Someone with PCOS might also have the following:
* LH:FSH ratio of 2:1 instead of 1:1
* Elevated estrogen levels
* Anxiety and/or depression
* Weight gain or difficulty losing weight, especially around the middle
* Elevated blood glucose levels or other markers of type 2 diabetes

Many women with PCOS will not have all of these symptoms, and some are asymptomatic, only diagnosed after difficulty conceiving. PCOS is not just a fertility problem. In fact, infertility is actually a side effect of PCOS, which is rooted in a metabolic condition caused by insulin resistance.

In healthy folks, insulin helps to make a gate for glucose (sugar) to pass through cell membranes where it will be processed into energy.

Insulin resistance develops due to high stress, unhealthy diet/lifestyle, or genetics; your body's cells reject insulin, so there is no way for the glucose to pass through.

For those with a predisposition to metabolic disorders, too many refined carbohydrates and sugars can trigger the cells to ignore the presence of insulin, demanding the body to make more and more insulin to "open the gate."

Glucose then floats around the bloodstream (elevating blood sugar) until it is converted to fat by the liver.

Insulin resistance also elevates insulin levels in the bloodstream. The excess insulin can stimulate the ovaries to produce large amounts of the male hormone testosterone. Excess testosterone quickly stimulates a bunch of follicles to grow right to the brink of maturation and then shuts down development. This results in the appearance of cysts, sometimes called a "ring of pearls," which are actually just immature follicles that never made it to lead follicle status.

In a healthy woman, during any given cycle, hundreds of follicles are recruited, with only one typically becoming the lead. In PCOS, follicles are recruited month after month, stimulated by testosterone, and abandoned before one is fully matured. Without a lead follicle, ovulation will not take place. Without ovulation, there is no progesterone, and hence, no luteal phase, leading to abnormal cycle progression. Anovulatory cycles can last weeks or months beyond the standard 28 days.

Every now and then, a lead follicle will emerge, resulting in ovulation. Once ovulation takes place, a woman with PCOS has just as much chance of becoming pregnant as another woman in her age group, though she may be at a higher risk for miscarriage due to hormone irregularities.

WESTERN MEDICAL TREATMENT OF PCOS

PCOS patients who wish to become pregnant need support with both ovulation and blood sugar control.

* **CLOMID (CLOMIPHENE CITRATE)** is a fertility drug often prescribed for PCOS patients, and it tends to work well in maturing follicles for ovulation.
* **CLOMID AND METFORMIN:** This combination stimulates the ovaries while controlling blood sugar levels.
* **GONADOTROPINS** are injectable drugs used to stimulate the ovaries. These drugs are used when Clomid alone is not creating the desired results or in an IVF cycle where Clomid is generally not strong enough to stimulate enough follicles to grow simultaneously.

PCOS patients who *do* not wish to get pregnant may be prescribed medications to control their symptoms, such as birth control pills to regulate their cycle, reduce testosterone and clear up acne, and/or diabetes medications to help control blood sugar and thereby reduce testosterone.

～ What the East Says ～

Because PCOS is a metabolic disorder, many patients with the syndrome will exhibit symptoms that practitioners of Chinese medicine would diagnose as Spleen deficiency, a.k.a. digestive weakness. Through maintaining a focus on improving diet and reducing insulin levels, the PCOS patient will start to feel better overall and may see signs of ovulation return, usually in the form of more regular menstrual cycles.

In addition to digestive weakness, patients who suffer from PCOS often have "damp" signs and symptoms including weight gain, sluggish metabolism, cystic ovaries, and cystic acne.

Along with diet and acupuncture, Chinese medicine uses herbal formulas to help regulate the menstrual cycle and control blood sugar. Phasic herbal protocols can be employed to assist the body in regulating the menstrual cycle and promoting ovulation. Treatment for PCOS will typically include the Kidney system (reproduction and the brain), the Spleen system (digestion), and the Liver/Gallbladder system (nervous system).

～ Diet and Lifestyle Considerations for PCOS ～

Conventional nutritional strategy for PCOS is simple: Because elevated blood sugar leads to a rise in insulin levels, which in turn causes higher testosterone levels, a low-glycemic

✳ PCOS AND WEIGHT GAIN ✳

Because of the actions of excess insulin, sugars tend to be shunted into either muscle cells where they are used for energy or fat cells where they are stored. Where they go is partially attributable to genetics, which may explain why some women with PCOS are overweight, while others are not. Regardless of weight gain, it is important for women with a PCOS diagnosis to regularly monitor their blood sugar levels to make sure they are not becoming more insulin resistant.

diet focused on real food is the PCOS patient's best friend.

Fats, proteins, and nonstarchy vegetables should be the mainstay of the PCOS fertility diet. Many women find a low-carb, grain-free, or Paleo diet to be the best solution for them.

Women with PCOS need to remember that their condition is, at its core, a metabolic condition, one that happens to interfere with ovulation. The most important thing a PCOS patient can do is to take steps to manage blood sugar through diet and supplements. In addition to a low-carb diet, supplements such as chromium picolinate, which helps control blood sugar, can be useful.

Perhaps just as important as diet is the need to exercise to manage blood sugar and control insulin levels. But don't overdo it if you're currently out of shape. Overtaxing your system may negate your efforts.

WHAT ABOUT DAIRY AND PCOS?

In traditional Chinese medicine, it is advised that women diagnosed with PCOS avoid dairy products because PCOS is thought to be a condition of "damp accumulation" and dairy generally contributes to this problem. As practitioners, we tend to take this on a case-by-case basis. For women who have dairy allergies or sensitivities, we certainly recommend avoiding milk, yogurt, cream, and cheese.

For others, we recommend only eating raw dairy from pasture-raised animals. Because of the natural probiotic content of raw milk products, they are often much easier for the body to assimilate, resulting in less damp and phlegm conditions.

✳ JENNY'S STORY ✳

Jenny, age 32, was trying to conceive her second child. She had a long history of PCOS and anovulatory cycles and was on day 40 since her last period. With the help of Chinese herbs and intensive dietary changes, Jenny ovulated 2 weeks into treatment and on day 53 of her cycle. Two weeks later she had a positive pregnancy test and went on to deliver a healthy boy.

Chapter 6

Thyroid Issues

THE THYROID GLAND IS A SMALL ORGAN LOCATED IN THE NECK that helps to manage the body's metabolism, blood calcium levels, and hormones. Imbalances of this organ can make conception a challenge. Thyroid health is a topic worthy of a book unto itself, so we've done our best to give you a useful starting point in this section.

∾ What the West Says: Hypothyroidism ∾

Hypothyroidism is a condition where an underactive thyroid fails to produce enough hormones, and various body systems slow down. Common symptoms can include fatigue, feeling cold, weight gain, sluggishness, depression, constipation, thinning hair, and irregular menstruation. For women trying to get pregnant, hypothyroidism may prevent ovulation or create irregular cycles including a shortened luteal phase. A shortened luteal phase can prevent implantation of a fertilized egg into the uterine wall, lead to miscarriage, or lead to decreased IQ in your future child if left unchecked during pregnancy.

Hypothyroidism is primarily diagnosed by checking blood levels of thyroid stimulating hormone (TSH). TSH is produced by the pituitary in response to a message from the hypothalamus that more thyroid hormone is needed by the body. TSH then tells the thyroid to make T4, which is then converted to an active form called T3.

While important, TSH is not the only component of blood to consider when evaluating thyroid function. While it's outside the scope of this book to go into the complex details of thyroid blood panels, if you have or suspect thyroid issues, be sure to have a complete thyroid workup from an experienced (and preferably integrative) endocrinologist or a holistic doctor.

Hypothyroidism commonly goes undiagnosed or underdiagnosed because the lab range for thyroid function is very wide—too wide in a lot of people's opinions (including ours). According to typical lab values, your thyroid is fine as long as it's at least between 0.5 and 5 miliU/L. If lower than 0.5, your diagnosis would be *hyperthyroid*, higher than 5, *hypothyroid*. That's because TSH is what stimulates the thyroid to produce hormones, so if there's not enough (hypo), more TSH will be required to give it a jump start; if there's too much (hyper), the reverse is true, and TSH will be very low.

From a fertility and pregnancy standpoint, a TSH of 5 is much too high. Most fertility specialists will recommend supplementation if your values come back above 2.5, and a level below 2 is ideal. You may have noticed that we aren't the "slap a Band-Aid on it" types of practitioners, but if you're racing the clock to make a baby, this might be one area to consider following biomedical advice. After you're through with childbearing, healing your metabolism and your thyroid are valiant and worthy undertakings, but the process can be lengthy. Synthetic thyroid hormone has been around a long time, and there are minimal side effects associated with short-term use for most patients.

For folks who don't tolerate synthetic thyroid hormone replacement (synthroid), are borderline, or simply prefer a more natural approach, other options do exist. Natural, desiccated forms of thyroid hormone include Armour Thyroid and Nature's Thyroid may be well tolerated when their synthetic counterpart is not. Keep in mind that most conventional MDs do not approve of bioidentical supplementation, so you may have an uphill battle—though one worth fighting, in our opinion.

∼ What the West Says: Hashimoto's Thyroiditis ⌣

Hashimoto's thyroiditis is an autoimmune condition, which occurs when the immune system creates antibodies that attack thyroid tissue. These antibodies lead to inflammation in the thyroid, resulting in decreased or impaired function. The same antibodies that attack the thyroid also attack the ovaries, so getting this condition under control is key for baby-making. In this case, Western medicine's only solution is to try to boost thyroid function by supplementing with synthetic thyroid hormone, with little to no solutions for getting the disease itself under control. Holistic medicine, on the other hand, has much more to offer when it comes to Hashimoto's.

~ What the West Says: Hyperthyroidism ~

Hyperthyroidism occurs when the thyroid becomes overactive. Rapid heartbeat, fatigue, weight loss, muscle weakness, irritability or anxiety, irregular menstruation, and infertility are some of its many symptoms.

Graves' disease is the most common cause of hyperthyroidism. Like Hashimoto's, Graves' is an autoimmune condition wherein antibodies produced by the immune system attack the thyroid gland and cause it to overproduce hormones.

Hyperthyroidism commonly affects women ages 20 to 40—just when fertility is of peak concern—and is particularly worrisome during pregnancy. Hyperthyroidism can be associated with a number of obstetric complications, including miscarriage and still birth, hyperemesis gravidarum (very severe/dangerous vomiting in pregnancy), low birth-weight babies, and other pregnancy complications, including preeclampsia.

The medicines used to treat hyperthyroid conditions are not ideal during pregnancy but may be necessary, because doing nothing can result in very poor outcomes for mom and baby. Women with a history of Graves' or hyperthyroidism should be monitored carefully throughout pregnancy to prevent the complications.

~ What the East Says ~

From a Chinese medicine perspective, thyroid hormone is Yang in nature. This is because it is responsible for the body's metabolic activity, which in and of itself is a Yang function. Nevertheless, all aspects of the body are balanced by both Yin and Yang, and when the scale is tipped, problems occur.

TREATING HYPOTHYROIDISM WITH CHINESE MEDICINE

When the thyroid becomes sluggish, Yang energy wanes, leading to typical Yang deficiency signs and symptoms including cold hands and feet, sluggish digestion, weight gain, depression, and irregular menstruation. Because of the thyroid's relationship to metabolism, there is a strong link between the thyroid and the Spleen/Stomach systems.

Herbs, acupuncture, and foods that warm the Yang; nourish the spleen and stomach; and boost Qi can often correct subtle thyroid imbalances, leading to the need for less medication and possibly reversal of a hypothyroid imbalance.

Thyroid issues are commonly linked to long periods of acute or chronic stress, which impacts the adrenal glands. Working on overcoming stress, supporting the adrenals with lifestyle and dietary choices, and making sure your body is well balanced in terms of minerals, antioxidants, and other key nutrients, is vital for a healthy endocrine system, including the thyroid.

TREATING HASHIMOTO'S WITH CHINESE MEDICINE

Because of the autoimmune component in Hashimoto's, one must look carefully at the Heart and Kidney systems (endocrine) along with the Spleen and Stomach (digestion/assimilation). Among their many other functions, the Heart and the Kidneys represent the balance between hormones and emotions and the nervous and endocrine system (hypothalamus/pituitary/thyroid/adrenals).

Working to balance these systems as well as treating the gut for digestive imbalances can help calm the immune system enough to stop the attack of thyroid tissue. Increased intake of certain antioxidants, including selenium and glutathione, are essential for reversing thyroid antibodies.

TREATING HYPERTHYROIDISM WITH CHINESE MEDICINE

Like the other side of a coin, hyperthyroidism in Chinese medicine is Yang energy gone wild. With excess Yang in the body, symptoms such as anxiety, insomnia, heart palpitations, and weight loss are predominant.

In this case, your Chinese medicine practitioner would look to provide you with herbs and acupuncture to cool you down by nourishing Yin and subduing Yang. Cooling foods should be the centerpiece of your diet. The same would essentially be true for Graves' disease, though the immune component would also be at play, much like a Hashimoto's diagnosis.

✳ ARE YOUR LINES OF COMMUNICATION OPEN?

Thyroid conditions are said to be a dysfunction of the throat chakra, the body's center for communication, creativity, connection, and personal intention. Resolving emotional issues related to these matters may also help improve thyroid conditions and minimize their impact on fertility.

∽ Diet and Lifestyle Considerations for Thyroid Disorders ∽

Thyroid function is complex and requires the presence and cooperation of many body functions and nutrients. Iodine, tyrosine, and selenium are a few key nutrients that the thyroid requires.

Iodine is a vital trace element that gets a bad rap in conventional circles. Nevertheless, iodine is essential for the production of thyroid hormones, as well as healthy breast and ovarian tissue. An iodine deficiency leads to an increase in TSH production, and elevated TSH can cause an enlargement of the thyroid, called goiter. Hashimoto's, genetics, and radiation can also cause goiter. Foods containing iodine should be regularly consumed in the case of hypothyroidism, including seaweed and ocean fish.

The amino acid tyrosine and the mineral selenium can help with hypothyroid and autoimmune thyroid symptoms such as low energy, poor focus, and lack of drive. Deficiency in both of these nutrients may be worse due to poor gut absorption.

There's plenty of advice out there to avoid foods that contain goitrogens to support thyroid health. Goitrogens are chemicals contained in foods such as broccoli, cauliflower, brussels sprouts, cabbage, sweet potatoes, and lima beans. It's our opinion that if you are getting enough thyroid-supporting nutrients in your diet—including adequate amounts of iodine, selenium, and tyrosine—then no compounds in foods considered goitrogenic are going to contribute to the enlargement of your thyroid gland. Focusing your energy on making sure your thyroid is functioning optimally (whether via Western medicine or holistic treatment) is a much better use of your time than avoiding broccoli.

People with Hashimoto's often have leaky gut syndrome and sensitivity to gluten, the protein found in wheat. The gluten molecule is also very similar to the protein molecule in dairy, called casein. People with Hashimoto's would do well to eliminate these foods from their diet until their antibodies are under control, and even then, should have them only sparingly.

Exercise plays a vital role in treating thyroid conditions. In the case of hypothyroidism, it can help by stimulating thyroid gland secretions and enhancing tissue sensitivity to the thyroid hormone. Exercise can relieve stress, and research shows that stress is often the main trigger for Graves' disease.

✳ JILL'S STORY ✳

Jill came in for an appointment after trying to conceive for almost a year. She was 34 and had a terribly high-stress job as a movie studio executive. Her menstrual cycles were long, often lasting 38 days or more. She complained of always feeling cold, especially in her hands and feet. She had some digestive issues and couldn't consume dairy without bloating and gas pain. Jill's TSH was 3.5—normal by standard lab values—and her T3 and T4 were normal.

Jill's protocol involved eliminating gluten and dairy from her diet completely, plus weekly acupuncture visits to stimulate her digestive function, thyroid, and overall endocrine system. She focused her diet on lots of real food, avoiding soy and raw food. She took herbs for fertility, and supplemented with antioxidants, including selenium and glutathione. After three months of treatment, her TSH was down to 2.2, and her periods were healthy and coming regularly every 30 to 32 days. She is working hard on managing the stress of her work-life balance and plans to resume her efforts to make a baby very soon.

Chapter 7

Unexplained Infertility

ONE OF THE MOST CHALLENGING FERTILITY OBSTACLES is when you are not getting pregnant month after month and there are not obvious reasons why. Thankfully, Chinese medicine can provide insight and potential solutions for unexplained infertility.

∼ What the West Says ∼

You've been trying to conceive for over a year with no luck.

Now you and your partner have had extensive hormone testing. Your partner's semen analysis indicates his sperm are healthy, plentiful, and champion swimmers. Your ultrasound shows a healthy uterus and ovaries. You've had an HSG test (hysterosalpingo-gram) and your fallopian tubes are open for business. For the most part, you menstruate and ovulate regularly. Everyone your age seems to be making babies left and right and you're still not pregnant. So what's the deal?

A diagnosis of unexplained infertility can be frustrating and sometimes devastating for couples trying to conceive. With no clear idea of what's delaying pregnancy, Western medicine offers very little hope for treatment, with many reproductive specialists simply recommending mounting interventions with each passing cycle.

∼ What the East Says ∼

Chinese medicine can offer sound explanations and effective solutions for otherwise unexplained infertility. Here are the most common causes of unexplained infertility from a Chinese medicine perspective:

INFERTILITY AS A NATURAL RESPONSE TO STRESS

While Chinese medicine can identify various causes based on your unique physiology, history, and lifestyle, the most common cause of unexplained infertility is stress. Whether it's from the continued frustration of not being able to conceive, confrontation with your boss, traffic, dental work, bills, or just a messy house—we all experience stress.

We've explained in detail on page 9 what happens to your body under stress. And while the stress reaction is both an essential and healthy human function, the problem with modern stressors is they tend to occur at a constant, low level, compared to the stress our ancestors experienced from the threat of being chased by a saber-toothed tiger. This means your body is all too often in a state of "fight or flight" and repeatedly being flooded with stress hormones.

If you're continually stressed out, you may be initiating a "normal" reaction to stress in your body: fertility shutdown. Stress hormones send a clear message to your body that it's not a good time to conceive. After all, why make a baby if you're about to be chomped by a mythical predator?

In addition to increased adrenaline and cortisol, stress can also deplete progesterone levels, leading to an imbalance between estrogen and progesterone, which can impair fertility. High cortisol levels are also associated with elevated prolactin, a hormone that can impair fertility by preventing ovulation.

High levels of stress can impede the free flow of Qi in the body. A woman with "Qi stagnation" will often suffer from migraines, digestive upset, PMS symptoms including irritability and painful breasts, and will have a unique quality to the pulse where it feels "wiry" like a guitar string. Sometimes the tongue will take on a dusky hue, reflecting stagnation in the body.

Once the Qi becomes sluggish or stuck, the blood circulation may also stagnate, resulting in painful, irregular menstrual cycles. Qi and Blood stagnation may also contribute to endometriosis, ovarian cysts, and uterine fibroids. Occasionally, women with Qi and Blood stagnation will not be aware of any symptoms, yet the stress continues to affect their bodies and fertility negatively.

THE BODY'S INABILITY TO HOLD A PREGNANCY

The same Qi that is responsible for healthy digestion also is responsible for the action of "holding and lifting" within the body. A deficiency or weakness in this Qi may result in bruising, varicosities, and hemorrhoids (the blood not being held within the vessels), prolapsed organs, fatigue, loose stools, gas, bloating, and cold extremities. A patient with this presentation may tend to gain weight on the lower half of her body (pear-shaped). If the lifting Qi is weak, the body doesn't have enough energy to carry a baby to term. Either miscarriage or inability to conceive may result.

A Chinese medicine practitioner can treat this pattern with herbs, acupuncture, diet, and lifestyle changes that strengthen the Qi, improve the digestion, and promote the body's ability to maintain a pregnancy.

INFERTILITY DUE TO WEAK REPRODUCTIVE ENERGY

Jing is reproductive energy and the genetic material we inherit from our parents. It's like a deep-pockets savings account of Qi that is not meant for daily spending. Jing controls all of the growth and development, reproductive function, and aging processes in the human body.

Some signs of declining Jing are sore and cold knees and/or lower back, a history of delayed onset of the menses, scanty blood flow during menses, low sex drive, fatigue, and frequent urination. Weak Essence can be caused by genetic inheritance, too much sex for men, too many pregnancies for a woman, or chronic overtaxing of energy by stress or poor diet and lifestyle. These patients may exhibit poor sperm or egg quality, high FSH, and an inability to conceive or carry a baby to term. If the Essence is weak and a baby comes to term, he or she may have developmental issues.

Though Western medicine tends to write off these patients as a lost cause due to "advanced maternal age," with consistent treatment, Chinese medicine can often help to reverse the effects of aging and increase the likelihood of successful conception and healthy pregnancy.

≈ How Chinese Medicine Can Help with Unexplained Infertility ≈

A diagnosis of unexplained infertility need not be a dead end on your road to parenthood. Acupuncture can harmonize and revitalize the body's Qi, improving circulation of Blood and energy to all vital organs. Most people find acupuncture to be a very relaxing experience, leaving you energized and better able to manage the stress in your life. Treatments can restore depleted Qi and help improve your reproductive potential. Your practitioner may also recommend herbal medicine and/or diet and lifestyle changes to help make your body a welcoming place to grow your baby.

Your commitment and participation will help to optimize the success of your treatments. Simple things such as what to eat, what to drink, stress levels, or how much to sleep can drastically affect egg quality during its 85-day journey to maturation, likelihood of successful fertilization, as well as the subsequent implantation and development.

✳ MARNI'S STORY ✳

Marni was 31 years old when she came into my office one October, after undergoing two IVF cycles to no avail. She was emotionally exhausted, feeling fearful and grief-stricken that she would never have a child of her own. Her fertility specialist said that her difficulties conceiving were unexplained, as her hormone levels were totally normal, she had a good number of antral follicles that responded well to stimulation drugs, and the embryos they produced were of good quality. She had been pregnant once, though the end result was a very early miscarriage, probably due to a genetic issue with the fetus.

Part of Marni's stress came from the need for fertility interventions at all. Always reliant on her intuition, she struggled with the notion that she couldn't conceive on her own. She decided to get off the fertility roller coaster for a while, continuing with weekly acupuncture, herbs, and paying extra attention to her already healthy, real food diet. She planned to continue through the holidays in this fashion, with plans to consider another IVF cycle in January.

Early in the new year, she came in for an appointment with a look of shock on her face. She had conceived naturally while on vacation with her husband over the holidays. Her beautiful son is now a toddler.

Chapter 8

The Male Factor

APPROXIMATELY 30 PERCENT OF INFERTILITY CASES ARE DUE TO SPERM ISSUES, also called male factor infertility. The most obvious indication of male infertility is a prolonged period of unprotected intercourse without conceiving a child. For most men, there are no obvious signs and symptoms, and the news that their swimmers are not top notch often comes as quite a shock.

∼ What the West Says ∽

Sometimes underlying problems such as genetic or structural issues that might prevent the passage of sperm, or hormone imbalances, come with signs and symptoms. These may include the following:
* Infertility, or the inability to conceive a child
* Erectile dysfunction or problems with ejaculation
* Loss of or reduction in facial or body hair (signifying hormonal imbalances)
* Pain, swelling, or lumps in or around the testicles
* Low sperm count, volume or motility, or poor morphology

Risk factors for sperm issues include the following:
* Using alcohol, tobacco, and certain illegal drugs
* Being overweight
* Having certain past or present infections
* Being exposed to toxins
* Overheating the testicles
* Having a prior vasectomy or vasectomy reversal
* Being born with a fertility disorder or having a blood relative with a fertility disorder

* Having certain medical conditions, including tumors and chronic illnesses
* Taking certain medications or undergoing medical treatments, such as surgery or radiation used for treating cancer
* Performing certain prolonged activities such as bicycling or horseback riding, especially on a hard seat or poorly adjusted bicycle

∾ When to Get a Semen Analysis ∾

In our experience, most men don't find out their sperm is less than superior until they've been trying to conceive for a while and their partners take it upon themselves to seek medical care: A semen analysis is part of the workup. Aside from any emotional stress involved, a semen analysis can never hurt, and it's not a bad idea to get things checked out *before* you start trying to make a baby.

Definitely get your swimmers assessed if you've been trying for a year or more and have any of the following:

* Pain, discomfort, swelling, or a lump in or around the testicles
* Erectile or ejaculation issues
* Lower than usual or a sudden decrease in sex drive
* A history of testicle or prostate issues
* A history of groin, testicle, penis, or scrotum surgery
* Reversed vasectomy (which can lead to development of antisperm antibodies where the immune system attacks the sperm)

SEMEN ANALYSIS RESULTS

Understanding the numbers on a sperm analysis can be confusing, especially because the parameters keep changing and there is more than one way of looking at them. Following is a comparison of the two most up-to-date perspectives, the Kruger Strict and the World Health Organization (WHO).

As you can see, the most recent (5th) edition from the WHO reduced the criteria for morphology from 14 to 4 percent. This is based on the addition of a test created by Dr. Kruger, who made the definition of normal form (morphology) MUCH stricter than it used to be. These forms are analyzed through a complex lab test.

What Kruger discovered is that sperm that meet the strict shape criteria have a better chance at making it through cervical mucus and up to the fallopian tube for fertilization. These more strict guidelines also seem to have improved IVF outcomes.

WHO Criteria for Normal Sperm

	5th edition	4th edition
Volume (mls)	1.5	2.0
Total Sperm (millions in ejaculate)	39	40
Sperm Concentration (millions per ml)	15	20
Total Motility	40	50
% Normal Forms	4	(14)

～ What the East Says ～

As we discussed earlier, genetics are the domain of the Kidneys, in particular Kidney Jing. Sperm themselves are essentially pure Jing, and thus problems with sperm quality or count are generally attributed to Kidney deficiency. Semen, a liquid substance, also has a yin component, so in the case of low overall volume, yin must be addressed. When Kidney deficiencies are compounded by obstructions, pain, or swelling, then a diagnosis of either Blood and Qi stagnation or damp heat is added on to the Kidney diagnosis.

Kidney deficiencies related to male fertility are diagnosed like this:

* **KIDNEY YIN DEFICIENCY** presents with erectile dysfunction and premature ejaculation, poor sperm morphology, low semen volume, possible overactive libido, restlessness, heat, and anxiety.
* **KIDNEY YANG DEFICIENCY** causes erectile dysfunction/inability to sustain erection, very low libido, low sperm count, poor motility, feeling cold, lethargy, and possibly depression.
* **DAMP HEAT** leads to swollen, hot, or painful genitals, pain with urination, and/or abnormal discharge from the penis.
* **QI AND BLOOD STAGNATION** are caused by congenital deformities (such as a missing vas deferens), undescended testicles, varicocele (a varicose vein in the scrotum), vasectomy, or other surgical history.

Much like his female counterpart's treatment, Chinese medicine practitioners address male infertility with herbs, acupuncture, diet, and lifestyle modifications. Because spermatogenesis takes roughly three months, it's a good idea to commit to implementing these changes for at least that long before expecting improvement to be reflected in new semen analysis.

～ Diet and Lifestyle for Improved Male Fertility ～

Pardon us for a moment while we completely generalize, but many men prefer NOT to talk and fuss about poor sperm quality and would rather take a handful of supplements than address their health with diet and lifestyle change. For those who are willing to focus on food, following a protocol rich in Jing foods combined with their Chinese medicine diagnosis is ideal.

When a quick and easy solution is as good as it's going to get, here is a list of general supplements for improving sperm quality and count. Take these daily, in addition to a customized herbal formula, to address any specific imbalances.

* Vitamin C with bioflavonoids—1,000 mg twice per day
* Vitamin E with mixed tocopherols—800 IU
* Selenium—200 to 400 mcg
* Zinc—60 mg per day (for sperm production and testosterone metabolism)
* Vitamin B_{12}—1,000 mg per day (promotes cell replication)
* L-arginine—4,000 mg (promotes cell replication)
* CoQ_{10}—200 mg (antioxidant)
* Acetyl L-carnitine—3 g (helps sperm motility)

✳ ROB'S STORY ✳

Rob, 34 years old, discovered he had a low sperm count and volume when attempting an IUI, so much so that they could not do the procedure. Aside from this discovery, Rob didn't have any particular health issues and was an easygoing guy, but he spent long hours working at his computer and lived a fairly sedentary lifestyle.

The couple opted to focus on a nutrient-dense fertility diet and eliminate grains and reduce sugar and dairy, as this was the best choice for his wife's condition. Rob noted that he was eating far less junk food with this new diet. He also started taking Chinese herbs, along with weekly acupuncture to focus on building Jing and Yin. Over the course of three months, his sperm count tripled and his volume also increased. They are now candidates for IUI again but are hoping to conceive naturally.

{ Part 4 }

Navigating the Medical Fertility World

At some point in your fertility journey, you may find yourself in need of help from a medical specialist. This experience will be much less intimidating if you're armed with a basic understanding of what tests you may need and why, as well as potential treatments that may be offered. If you're unsure about whether or not you should seek medical care, please read Building a Strong Support Team on page 41.

One thing to remember when it comes to lab values and other diagnostic tests: These results show a snapshot of the past, not your potential. Don't feel doomed by less than stellar results. Consider "irregularities" as helpful information and make changes to how you're living and decisions regarding treatment accordingly.

Chapter 1

Understanding the Basic Fertility Workup

A BLOOD TEST THAT MEASURES HORMONE VALUES is vitally important for diagnosing causes of fertility challenges. The following are checked to evaluate a person's likelihood of becoming pregnant and having a healthy child:

* Estradiol (the component of estrogen related to reproduction)
* FSH (follicle stimulating hormone)
* LH (luteinizing hormone)
* TSH (thyroid stimulating hormone)
* AMH (anti-Müllerian hormone)
* Progesterone
* Prolactin

In addition to these levels, testosterone and other "male" hormones may be evaluated, along with a glucose/metabolic panel if PCOS is suspected.

∼ Estradiol (E2) ∽
•••

E2 is the component of estrogen produced by the follicles in your ovaries. The level of E2 in your blood is the lowest at the onset of your period (because the eggs are just barely beginning to develop and secrete estradiol), and this is when it must be checked to be diagnostically meaningful (day 2 or 3 at the latest).

Estradiol levels naturally rise as your body selects a "lead" follicle for that cycle and continues to rise as the follicle progresses toward maturity and ovulation around day 14.

On cycle day 2 or 3, the range for E2 is roughly 20 to 70 pg/ml. Because of the relationship between E2 and FSH, abnormally high levels on cycle day 2 could be suppressing the true FSH value. Generally, high day 2 estradiol values are caused by a functional cyst (a follicle from the previous cycle that didn't ovulate properly), polycystic ovary syndrome (PCOS), or pregnancy.

≈ Follicle Stimulating Hormone (FSH) ≈

FSH is a hormone released by the pituitary when the hypothalamus tells it that it's time to recruit a new lead follicle for the cycle that's just starting. Because FSH is lowest on cycle day 2 or 3, it must be checked at this time to have any clinical relevance.

As we age, FSH levels will start to rise earlier, even before the period starts, leading to an early lead follicle. This may be due to decreasing egg quality and quantity (which means they aren't releasing as much estradiol as they once were).

Up until recently, FSH was the primary predictor of ovarian reserve, which is one of the indicators for the likelihood of achieving a healthy pregnancy. Today, AMH (see below) is also used to diagnose ovarian reserve.

FSH ranges are as follows (ranges can vary from lab to lab; this is a generalization):
* Ideal: 4 to 9
* Okay: 9 to 11
* Less than ideal: 11 to 13
* Poor prognosis: 14 and higher

It is important to understand that these numbers are primarily used to determine whether or not a woman is likely to respond to the medications used in fertility treatments because those medications mimic the same actions as FSH on the developing follicles. Basically, they are synthetic FSH. So, if a woman's follicles are not responding to her own intrinsic FSH, then she is likely to be a poor responder to fertility drugs. It's also important to note that FSH levels can vary from month to month, so don't be too discouraged if your numbers are slightly elevated—they may very well come down.

High FSH does not mean that you cannot become pregnant naturally, especially when lifestyle and dietary modifications are practiced for several months. There are countless cases of women becoming pregnant with high FSH levels, so don't get discouraged if this is your situation. Lowering FSH levels is an area where herbs and acupuncture really shine. If high FSH levels are standing between you and an IVF cycle, think about finding yourself a fertility acupuncturist right away.

∼ AMH (Anti-Müllerian Hormone) ∼

AMH is secreted by the granulosa cells in the ovary. This hormone is what holds back potential follicles from ovulation so that humans do not naturally breed litters of children. Thus, as ovarian reserve declines, AMH levels go down correspondingly.

AMH numbers decline with age and are used to predict ovarian reserve along with FSH. Low AMH does not necessarily indicate poor egg quality, especially if it is low in a younger woman. Unlike FSH, AMH levels do not predict an individual's probable response to IVF medications; AMH predicts ovarian potential. AMH levels can be checked at any point in the cycle.

∼ Luteinizing Hormone (LH) ∼

LH is secreted by the pituitary gland when the growing egg signals the brain that it is mature and ready to ovulate. At this point in the cycle, an LH surge occurs, sending a significant amount of LH down to the ovaries, leading to ovulation.

Typically, this hormone is tested on day 2 and is usually in about a 1:1 ratio with FSH. A 2:1 ratio is one indicator of possible PCOS, but it's not diagnostic without considering other factors.

LH also plays a role in the conversion of the follicle to a corpus luteum, the outer shell of the follicle which produces progesterone during the second half of the menstrual cycle and into the first trimester, should pregnancy occur.

∼ Thyroid Stimulating Hormone (TSH) ∼

TSH is secreted by the pituitary in order to stimulate the thyroid to produce T4 and T3. The thyroid helps to manage the body's metabolism, blood calcium levels, and hormones, and an imbalanced thyroid will often contribute to fertility issues.

The normal reference ranges for thyroid disease are too broad for pregnancy. While the "normal" range for thyroid is measured by a TSH of 1 to 5, most functional medical doctors and fertility specialists prefer to see the level below 2.5.

If you are symptomatic for a thyroid condition and your TSH is normal, it is important to request further testing, including a complete thyroid panel that measures all the components of T3 and T4 as well as checking for thyroid antibodies that could indicate an autoimmune condition such as Graves' disease or Hashimoto's thyroiditis. See page 174 for a detailed summary of thyroid function.

∼ **Progesterone** ∽

Progesterone is a hormone mainly secreted by the corpus luteum during the second half of the menstrual cycle. During this time, progesterone thickens the uterine lining, called the endometrium, in preparation for possible implantation.

Progesterone causes a slight rise in body temperature and is the reason for the rise in temperature seen on BBT charts just after ovulation has occurred, as well as maintaining these higher temperatures throughout the second half of the cycle (luteal phase) and throughout pregnancy. If progesterone levels are too low following ovulation, an otherwise healthy pregnancy could result in miscarriage.

Progesterone levels are typically checked about five days following ovulation. Ideally, the value will be above 10 ng/ml, an indication that ovulation has occurred and the corpus luteum is doing its job. Progesterone levels generally decline with age, and low progesterone can be a sign of improper ovulation.

Low levels are often supplemented with synthetic progesterone—usually in the form of vaginal suppositories or injections—to ensure that a potentially healthy pregnancy isn't derailed by a lackluster corpus luteum.

∼ **Prolactin** ∽

Prolactin is a hormone secreted by the pituitary. Its primary function is to promote lactation after a baby is born. Prolactin is not cycle day dependent and can thus be checked at any point.

High levels of prolactin (over 25 ng/ml) inhibit estrogen production, which is why a lactating woman often won't ovulate or menstruate until she stops or dramatically reduces her breastfeeding.

While uncommon, it is possible to have high prolactin levels in the absence of lactation. This is typically caused by a benign tumor on the pituitary, called a prolactinoma, which wreaks havoc on normal hormone secretion and can interfere with ovulation and estrogen levels (among other things). Elevated prolactin can also be caused by stress, hypothyroid, kidney disease, and some medications.

Prolactin levels will naturally fluctuate throughout the day and rise after eating or sexual activity. If your prolactin levels are high, it's important to recheck them in the morning while fasting and with no sex the day before.

Depending on the severity, this condition may be treated with a drug called bromocriptine, or in a worst-case scenario, with surgery to remove the benign tumor.

∼ Day 2/3 Ultrasound ∼

Each month, our ovaries mature hundreds (and up to a thousand or so) eggs, only one of which will become the "lead" follicle, set on the road to ovulation. When planning an IVF or medicated IUI cycle, your doctor will likely perform an ultrasound on the second day of your cycle to see how many follicles (called antral follicles) are visible.

The importance of the ultrasound happening on day 2 resides in the likelihood that a lead follicle won't have been recruited yet, providing a level playing field for all of the visible antral follicles to respond to ovarian stimulation medications. "Synchronized" follicles on day 2 offer the best chance for a successful IVF cycle.

A high antral follicle count (12 to 15 or more) is a good indication that you will respond well to IVF medications, whereas a low count (less than 5) is a signal that your eggs might not respond very well. An intermediate response (6 to 12) is less predictable. Keep in mind that age plays a huge role in follicle health, so lower numbers in a younger woman still may bode well.

Ultrasounds can also be used on any day of the cycle to observe ovarian health, make a preliminary assessment of the uterine cavity, and check ovarian reserve.

∼ The HSG Test: Are the Pipes Clear and the Walls Smooth? ∼

The hysterosalpingogram (HSG) is a baseline test given to women experiencing fertility challenges in order to assess the inner walls of the uterus and the patency (openness) of the fallopian tubes.

The test is performed through the insertion of a catheter through the cervix and into the uterus. Radiopaque dye, similar to that used in an angiogram (or other such procedure), is then squirted into the uterus and through the fallopian tubes. If the tubes are open, it will be apparent to the radiologist, as the dye goes into the tubes via the uterus and cascades out the other end.

The HSG also looks at the inner walls of the uterus, in order to rule out certain abnormalities that could potentially impede or prevent implantation or compete for blood supply with a developing fetus. These include things such as fibroids, polyps, and uterine septum. On occasion, this test can be curative as well as diagnostic, as it may actually clear a fallopian obstruction, thus allowing for easier progression of a fertilized embryo down the tube toward its uterine destination.

Most women report this test to be uncomfortable, and the use of some type of relaxant such as valium may be recommended.

～ The Semen Analysis ～

Thirty percent or more of couples experiencing infertility have male factor issues. Either the **quantity** (volume, concentration, or count), **quality** (morphology or DNA issues), or **motility** (strength and directionality) are compromised. Sometimes, all three are an issue. Rarely, there are no sperm at all, a condition called azoospermia.

In 2010 the WHO updated its parameters for a normal sperm analysis. Based on those changes, a healthy sperm profile will look like this:

Volume	1.5 ml
Concentration	20 million/ml
Progressive motility	60%
Normal forms (morphology)	>4%

Remember: Today's sperm started its road to maturation roughly 90 days ago. Anything significant, including a high fever, extreme stress, excessive hot tub use, wearing snug pants frequently, or physical activity that could hinder sperm health (such as long-distance biking) should be considered and modified if the numbers are unfavorable. It's a good idea to recheck sperm a few times before arriving at a diagnosis.

～ Postcoital Testing ～

Throughout a woman's cycle, her cervix produces fluid, which changes based on where she is in relation to ovulation. In the days just after the period, there is a slow increase in cervical mucus, which culminates in a slippery, egg white–like substance around the time of ovulation.

This fluid makes vaginal pH more hospitable to sperm making it easier for the sperm to swim through the cervix.

Occasionally, cervical mucus doesn't lend itself to assisting the sperm during ovulation and can even prevent it from getting past the gate at all.

Postcoital testing is done by instructing a couple to have intercourse during the window of ovulation and then having them come in to the doctor within 12 hours. A sample is taken from the woman's vagina and looked at under a microscope. If viable sperm are visualized, all is well. If all of the sperm are dead, it indicates a cervical factor.

Some of the reasons for cervical factor infertility include a history of HPV or surgery such as a cone biopsy. Also, an overactive immune system may create antisperm antibodies; essentially her body thinks the sperm is a harmful pathogen rather than a friendly invader.

Chapter 2
....

Insemination—IUI and ICI

INTRAUTERINE INSEMINATION (IUI) AND INTRACERVICAL INSEMINATION (ICI) are procedures where sperm is injected into a woman's uterus (IUI) or cervix (ICI) to increase her odds of becoming pregnant by bypassing the treacherous cervix, giving the sperm a considerable leg up on their journey.

ICI is much less effective than IUI, and it is rarely performed in fertility clinics these days. Some women attempt an at-home version of insemination (ICI), particularly if they are otherwise fertile, but require donated sperm due to sexual orientation or single parenthood.

IUI is typically done under the supervision of an OB-GYN or fertility specialist (RE). This can be done with a woman's natural cycle or with medical stimulation.

≈ Natural IUI ≈
● ●

This protocol has a woman monitor herself for ovulation. A sperm sample is given and typically washed to improve its overall viability. A catheter full of sperm is then threaded into the uterus.

≈ Medicated/Stimulated IUI ≈
● ●

These cycles are performed after administering medications to a woman to stimulate multiple follicles at once, thus maximizing her chances of having a healthy egg at the time of conception. Medicated IUI cycles are ideally performed under strict monitoring to ensure the ovaries are continuing to respond favorably and to avoid the risk of multiples, overstimulating the ovaries (OHSS), and "overcooking" the eggs, which renders them useless.

Once the follicles are ready to go, a trigger shot of HCG is given to facilitate ovulation. HCG (human chorionic gonadotropin) has a molecular makeup very similar to LH, the hormone that surges just before ovulation. It takes roughly 36 hours from the time of the trigger shot for ovulation to occur, so IUIs are typically scheduled to accommodate this time frame.

Chapter 3

IVF and Other Advanced Fertility Treatments

IVF, OR IN VITRO FERTILIZATION, is a method for increasing a patient's fertility odds by:

* Increasing the number of follicles available in a given cycle to maximize the chances of achieving pregnancy
* Assisting with the fertilization of mature eggs through procedures such as ICSI (intra-cytoplasmic sperm injection) and assisted hatching
* Allowing for genetic testing of embryos to eliminate any which are not chromosomally normal (PGD or PGS)
* Circumventing tubal issues
* Overcoming sperm issues

IVF should always be performed by a board certified reproductive endocrinologist/infertility specialist—at a reputable clinic with a highly regarded laboratory. Take the time to find out which office has the best reputation in your area, and don't shy away from spending a little extra for the best clinic you can find. The cost of having to undergo multiple cycles due to physician mistakes is not worth the money saved in the long run. That's not to say it will work the first time you try at a reputable clinic, but you want to hedge your bets wherever possible, and in this case, you get what you pay for.

It is important to remember that IVF is merely a strategy for maximizing an individual's fertility *wherever* it is in that moment. **IVF is not a cure for infertility,** especially when it is due to advanced maternal age or severely compromised sperm. As we get older, our eggs are more and more likely to divide abnormally, which leads to problems such as Down syndrome. While IVF does increase the number of chances you and your partner get in a cycle to create a healthy embryo, it has no impact on whether or not the embryos will actually cooperate and divide normally. That doesn't mean it won't help, or even significantly increase your odds of achieving a healthy pregnancy, but it's not magic.

When taken at face value, IVF success rates can seem pretty dismal. However, keeping in mind that a healthy couple in their prime reproductive years has roughly a 1 in 5 (20 percent) chance at pregnancy in a given cycle can lend a little bit of perspective to projected IVF outcomes.

Here are the success rates for live birth outcomes for IVF in the United States, according to the American Pregnancy Association:

* 30 to 35 percent for women under age 35
* 25 percent for women ages 35 to 37
* 15 to 20 percent for women ages 38 to 40
* 6 to 10 percent for women over age 40

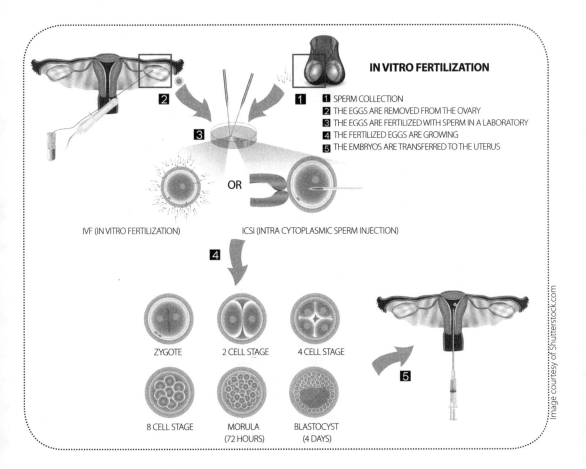

IN VITRO FERTILIZATION

1 SPERM COLLECTION
2 THE EGGS ARE REMOVED FROM THE OVARY
3 THE EGGS ARE FERTILIZED WITH SPERM IN A LABORATORY
4 THE FERTILIZED EGGS ARE GROWING
5 THE EMBRYOS ARE TRANSFERRED TO THE UTERUS

IVF (IN VITRO FERTILIZATION)

ICSI (INTRA CYTOPLASMIC SPERM INJECTION)

ZYGOTE

2 CELL STAGE

4 CELL STAGE

8 CELL STAGE

MORULA
(72 HOURS)

BLASTOCYST
(4 DAYS)

~ The IVF Cycle ~

Following is a brief overview of each step in the IVF cycle. If you are considering this type of treatment, you will of course go over all of these phases in detail with your doctor.

DAY 2 TESTS

On day 2 of the menstrual period, a woman goes into the fertility office to have her E2/FSH levels drawn. She also undergoes a transvaginal ultrasound to count and measure the number of antral follicles (the ones that are candidates for responding to the medications).

In an optimal cycle, all of the potential follicles should be about the same size. If one follicle is already bigger than the rest (a lead follicle), then the cycle should be delayed until the next month. An early lead follicle will absorb a disproportionate amount of medication and result in a less than ideal outcome. Don't let impatience get the best of you here. It's best to wait until the conditions are optimal than rush ahead.

MEDICATION START

Once the lab results are in (later on day 2) and the follicles are confirmed synchronized, IVF medications are self-administered via injection, usually starting that very evening. It is critical to follow instructions to a tee and to call the office if you have any questions or concerns. Getting off track could sabotage the cycle.

CHECK-IN

After a few days of injections, the patient returns to the clinic to check for progress via ultrasound and blood work. It is expected that E2 levels continue to rise with each passing day, as the developing follicles are continuing to secrete more and more estrogen as they grow.

Cycles that become significantly desynchronized may be canceled at any time, though some doctors will push through and allow the larger follicles to become over-mature in an effort to save the smaller majority. We personally find this practice to be problematic, as it is often the larger "lead" follicles that are the most likely to be healthy. Once again, patience is key, and it's better to wait it out for an ideal cycle.

The process of self-administering medications typically lasts 10 to 12 days, with frequent visits to the doctor for monitoring and blood work. Once the RE determines that the follicles are at the peak of their maturity (measured by E2 levels), then an HCG trigger shot is administered, roughly 36 hours before retrieval.

EGG RETRIEVAL

Follicle aspiration (retrieval) is a minor surgical procedure, which is performed by an RE in order to remove all of the developed follicles from a woman's ovaries for fertilization in the lab. The procedure is performed in a sterile operating room under heavy sedation (she will be asleep), by inserting an ultrasound-guided needle through the wall of the vagina and into the ovaries, one side at a time. The RE skillfully suctions the follicles and surrounding fluid out of the ovaries, and they are immediately assessed for maturity.

Once the procedure is over, the follicles are taken to the lab where they are stripped of their outer membrane to reveal the single-celled ova and then fertilized with her partner's sperm, or donor sperm—from a sample given that same morning—or from a frozen sample.

FERTILIZATION

Ova are fertilized one of two ways: naturally or via ICSI.

NATURAL FERTILIZATION is the process whereby sperm and egg are placed together in a petri dish and left to fertilize on their own. This method allows for "natural selection" to occur.

ICSI (intracytoplasmic sperm injection) is the process whereby a single sperm is corralled into a pipette and skillfully injected into the ova's cytoplasm. This procedure is typically performed when a man's sperm parameters are poor, in order to increase the odds of having a healthy sperm meet the egg.

The day following retrieval and fertilization (considered day 1 in IVF terms), the follicles are assessed. Normally fertilized ova will have two nuclei and are referred to as 2PNs (two pronuclei). If a "freeze all" cycle was planned, embryos are often frozen at this stage because this gives them the highest thaw rate. If a fresh cycle is occurring, then the 2PNs are left to continue growing for two to four more days. Embryos can also be frozen as day 5 (or sometimes day 6) blastocysts, if there any left over at the time of transfer.

EMBRYO TRANSFER

Embryo transfer usually occurs on either day 3 (cleavage stage) or day 5 (blastocyst stage). The choice between these two days is related to how many embryos there are to choose from, how old the mother-to-be is, or clinic preference.

Many clinics routinely do day 3 transfers, while others feel that day 5 offers better results. The difference in development between a day 3 embryo and a day 5 blastocyst is considerable. Typically, there is an attrition rate of roughly 50% or more during these two days. What this means is that embryos that are not chromosomally normal or are otherwise compromised won't make it through the complex cell dividing that must take place to go from the four-to-eight-cell embryo stage to the hundred-plus-cell blastocyst stage. Hence, it is presumed that embryos that survive to the blastocyst stage have a greater chance of being chromosomally normal than their day 3 counterparts.

For this reason, significantly fewer blastocysts are transferred on day 5 than embryos on day 3. The decision of how many to transfer is between a couple and her doctor, and should take into account her age, past cycles, and guidelines put forth by the ASRM (American Society of Reproductive Medicine).

Here are the ASRM recommendations by age for number of embryos to transfer:

* **Under 35:** one embryo for favorable prognosis/blastocyst transfer; one or two embryos for favorable prognosis/cleavage-stage transfer; two embryos for all others
* **35 to 37 years:** two embryos for all patients; three embryos for women with less favorable prognoses who receive cleavage-stage embryos
* **38 TO 40 years:** two embryos for favorable prognosis/blastocyst transfer; four embryos for less favorable prognosis/cleavage-stage transfer; three embryos for all others
* **41 to 42 years:** three embryos for those receiving blastocysts; five embryos for those receiving cleavage-stage embryos

The procedure for transferring embryos is quite simple, especially when compared to the complexities of the rest of the IVF cycle. Mom-to-be is placed on an exam table, in the same position she would be in for a Pap smear. A speculum is inserted and her cervix is cleaned off with the same media that are currently housing her embryos. Next, a catheter is inserted into the cervix, and threaded to about 1 cm (approximately half an inch) from the top (fundus) of her uterus. Then, a thin, flexible catheter containing the embryos for transfer is inserted through the already placed catheter and threaded to the top of the uterus as well. At this point, the embryos are pushed gently into the cervix, at the optimal spot for healthy implantation to occur.

In order to guide the catheter to its ideal location, ultrasound is typically used on the abdomen. Usually, a woman is asked to drink plenty of water prior to transfer so that her bladder will help to flatten out the uterus, making it easier for the doctor to find the ideal location. Most women find that the full bladder sensation is the most uncomfortable aspect of embryo transfer.

Following transfer, a woman is usually left to rest for 15 to 60 minutes and then released to go home for a day or so of modified bed rest (some clinics recommend much longer periods of rest).

One of the greatest fears that couples have following embryo transfer is that their newly placed embryos will somehow fall out when she stands up. This definitely won't happen. First, the uterus is not on a vertical plane, and second, the inside of the uterus is cavernous, with lots of ridges that can catch an embryo where it lands. One of the clinics we work with very frequently allows patients to get up to relieve themselves immediately following transfer, without any compromise to their pregnancy rates. So, worry not. If it's a healthy embryo, standing up won't ruin your chances.

THE TWO-WEEK WAIT AND PREGNANCY TESTS

Finally, the two-week wait begins. During this time, blood work may be done to make sure that the patient's body has enough estrogen and progesterone to ensure pregnancy can be sustained. At last, about 14 days following retrieval, blood work is done to check for HCG in the bloodstream. A number above 50 confirms pregnancy, but lower numbers can sometimes catch up. Very low numbers indicate a likely chemical pregnancy, which means that while implantation did occur, the embryo is not growing. Follow-up blood work will confirm whether or not a pregnancy is chemical or viable.

When a positive pregnancy is confirmed, blood work is generally done every few days to ensure a healthy rise in HCG levels until six to seven weeks gestation, when an ultrasound is performed to check for a fetal heartbeat. A healthy rise in HCG is indicated by numbers that double every other day—if it goes up even more than that, it's a good thing.

Patients will generally stick with their fertility specialist through about the eight-week mark, at which point they are "graduated" to their OB-GYN or midwife of choice. In the case of high-risk factors or multiples, your RE might want you to see a high-risk perinatologist.

∼ Chinese Medicine Can Support IVF ∽

Chinese medicine has been used for thousands of years to help regulate the reproductive systems in men and women. While it is quite difficult to draw exact parallels between Eastern and Western medical models, we can hypothesize how the mechanisms of acupuncture, in particular, may influence a woman's fertility in the following ways:

* Affecting neurotransmitters, which in turn influences the menstrual cycle, ovulation, and fertility by increasing the release of gonadotropin-releasing hormones (the stuff that your hypothalamus sends to your pituitary to tell it what to do, such as release FSH)
* Improving blood flow to the uterus, by reducing the amount of uterine sympathetic (fight-or-flight pathway) nerve activity
* Stimulating the release of endorphins (opioids that your brain makes), which directly inhibits the stress response

The Manheimer study, published in the *British Medical Journal*, evaluated whether acupuncture improves the rates of pregnancy and live birth on women undergoing IVF. The data looked at 1,366 women undergoing IVF and concluded that **acupuncture given with IVF does indeed improve pregnancy rates in a way that is both significant and clinically relevant.**

Yet another study from the *Journal of Alternative and Complementary Medicine* analyzed 1,069 women undergoing IVF (using their own eggs on a fresh cycle). The researchers concluded that a combination of herbs, acupuncture, nutrition, and lifestyle changes, termed "Whole System Traditional Chinese Medicine," dramatically reduced biochemical pregnancies and improved live birth rates by 77 percent.

ACUPUNCTURE AND IVF

The Paulus study, published in 2002 in the *Journal of Fertility and Sterility*, looked at the effects of acupuncture on pregnancy rates when it was performed immediately before and after embryo transfer. The results were impressive, increasing the presence of a fetal sac at six weeks gestation from 26.3 percent in the non-acupuncture control group to 42.5 percent in the group who received acupuncture. That's a 16.1 percent difference, which is quite clinically significant in IVF-land. More studies are being published every year, confirming the powerful impact of Chinese medicine on fertility.

Beyond treatment directly supporting the embryo transfer, we see patients in the days between egg retrieval and embryo transfer to help detox the body from all those medications and prepare the uterus for implantation. We also see patients three to five days after embryo transfer to assist with implantation and at least one more time to help ease worry during the dreaded two-week wait.

While we look to studies for validation that our work is providing meaningful clinical results, the true test of the benefits of incorporating Chinese medicine, a healthy diet, and appropriate herbs and supplements into your life is YOU. The fertility journey can be fraught with unexpected hairpin turns. Your ability to cope with the ups and downs of the ride is fully dependent on your physical, emotional, and mental state. Not to mention the untold benefits to your future offspring who will depend on you for every cell in their bodies once conception occurs.

The value of making the necessary lifestyle changes while trying to conceive are not just reflected in the increased statistical outcomes of using Chinese medicine, they are reflected in the way you get through each day with adequate sleep, abundant energy, and a positive outlook. We are not saying that every day will be filled with unicorns and butterflies, but we can say for sure that bringing your entire being into balance will make the journey much smoother.

HERBS, SUPPLEMENTS, AND IVF

Generally speaking, we don't prescribe Chinese herbs during IVF because no one wants to risk any interactions that could interfere with progress. In reality, it is sometimes appropriate to consider using herbs during IVF, especially if it isn't your first cycle, you're on the older side, or you have a complicated medical condition. The bottom line is that you should NEVER self-prescribe herbal medicines during IVF treatments, you should work with a qualified Chinese medical fertility specialist, and your RE should be aware of what you are doing.

In terms of supplements, whatever you plan to do for prenatal nutrition (whether a focused, food-based approach or a supplement), it is ideal to be well into the routine of it for at least three months before conception.

Aside from Chinese herbs, other supplements commonly used during IVF include coenzyme Q_{10} and DHEA. CoQ_{10} is an antioxidant touted for its benefits to heart health. Some studies have suggested that CoQ_{10} can increase the amount of mitochondria (the cell's powerhouse) in the ovaries, which could make cell division more successful when an egg is fertilized.

DHEA is a hormone made by the adrenals that is the precursor to testosterone, the building block of estrogen. Side effects from DHEA can include increased body odor and acne. Women with PCOS should steer clear of DHEA.

As with anything taken during this time, be sure to check with your medical support team (RE, acupuncturist, etc.).

✳ MINI FERTILITY CLEANSE FOR WOMEN UNDERGOING MEDICATED FERTILITY TREATMENTS ✳

After all of the injections and hormones of an IVF (or medicated IUI) cycle, the three to five days between egg retrieval and embryo transfer can serve as a great opportunity for a very gentle cleanse.

Think of this as your chance to clear your body of anything it doesn't need, making way for implantation in fertile ground.

If your partner isn't one for helping in the kitchen, we recommend that you make bone broth and Bieler's Broth (page 105 to 106) ahead of retrieval so it's ready to serve when you get home by the eve of your transfer.

Note that if you are doing a "day 5 transfer," continue with variations of days 2 and 3 until the morning of your transfer. *(continued on next page)*

✳ DAY 1 (DAY OF RETRIEVAL) ✳

Clear heat and toxicity, nourish Jing and Blood, activate Qi, and warm the Uterus

FOLLOWING YOUR PROCEDURE, drink a cup (235 ml) of hot water with the juice of half a lemon, a pinch of cayenne, and a teaspoon of honey to help cleanse the liver and heal from your procedure.

LUNCH (OR WHENEVER YOU'RE HUNGRY): Bieler's Broth (page 105), made with bone broth instead of water

SNACKS (ANY TIME THROUGHOUT THE DAY): Freshly squeezed or pressed green juice with ginger; cut-up veggies; apples; chicken broth seasoned to your liking; Bieler's Broth (page 105); Fertility Tea (page 118)

DINNER: Roasted chicken (use the bones to make more broth) with sautéed veggies (broccoli, asparagus, zucchini, etc.), cooked in coconut oil or butter and roasted sweet potato with butter

✳ DAY 2 ✳

Clear heat and toxicity, activate Qi, and nourish Jing and Blood

BREAKFAST: Hot water with lemon and honey (cayenne if you'd like); fruit salad (whatever is in season); and soft-boiled eggs (or eggs any way)

LUNCH: Bieler's Broth (page 105) or leftovers from dinner, or a mason jar salad

SNACKS: Same as Day 1

DINNER: Quinoa, soaked at least 8 hours and cooked in bone broth; and veggies sautéed in coconut oil

✳ DAY 3 ✳

Nourish Jing and Blood, and clear heat and toxicity

BREAKFAST: Hot water with lemon and honey (no cayenne); boiled eggs; and fruit

LUNCH: Sweet potato with butter; mason jar salad with chicken

DINNER: Bacon Tomato Quiche with Cauliflower Crust (page 94); and Wilted Dandelion Greens with Lemon and Feta (page 117)

✳ DAY 4 (DAY OF TRANSFER) ✳

Nourish Jing and Blood, and soothe the nervous system

BREAKFAST: Hot water with lemon and honey and Creamy Egg Drop Soup (page 95)

LUNCH: Leftover Bacon Tomato Quiche with Cauliflower Crust (page 94)

DINNER: Magical Chili (page 96) and a simple salad

SNACKS: Green juice with ginger or Fertility Tea (page 118)

∾ Exercise and IVF ∾

While we believe moderate exercise is a very important part of a balanced lifestyle, there are times when you have to hold back for your own safety. IVF medications that stimulate your ovaries to produce multiple follicles can result in ovarian swelling. This "swelling" occurs along a spectrum from mildly bloated to terribly uncomfortable, depending on how much medication you receive and how responsive your ovaries are to it.

One of the risks with IVF stimulation is a condition called ovarian hyperstimulation syndrome (OHSS), wherein the ovaries become very enlarged, heavy, and painful. There is also small risk associated with exercise during this time that could result in a twist (torsion) in your fallopian tubes—something you definitely want to avoid.

Ovarian torsion is very painful and extremely serious, which is why the general recommendation is to lay low while the follicles are on the rise. Walking is usually fine, unless true OHSS is at hand, in which case you may have to tread very lightly until things settle down again. In severe cases of true OHSS, it can take several months to resolve.

Your fertility specialist will likely tell you to avoid all vigorous exercise from the start of medications through your pregnancy test, and we suggest you heed this advice. Gentle walks outdoors are fine, and we highly encourage them, especially if you can get out in nature for a while. Meditation, prayer, breath work, and journaling are all great stress busters to double up on while exercise is off-limits.

··

Chapter 4

Other Options—
Sperm Donation, Egg
Donation, Surrogacy,
and Adoption

PERHAPS THE MOST DIFFICULT DECISION to be made on the journey toward parent-hood is when to stop pursuing having a biological child. Moving on to some type of third-party parenthood—whether it be sperm or egg donation, surrogacy or adop-tion—requires closure, and for many couples, comes with a great deal of grief. While this decision is ultimately very personal, there are a few things to consider as you make your way toward the ultimate goal of having a family of your own.

Before we break these down, let's spend a minute talking about DNA. According to the Human Genome Project, 99.9 percent of human DNA is identical from person to person. That leaves a mere 0.1 percent to account for the differences between us. Genetically speaking, that is. While we don't want to minimize the anguish that comes with choosing to move on from one's own biological material to donated material, let's keep in mind just how much we are alike when it comes to our DNA.

Epigenetics, on the other hand, are much more a function of the way an individual's environment influences who they become as they travel through life. Everything from diet to growing up in a functional family, getting a good education, and feeling loved and protected will influence which *aspects* of our genes express themselves as we age. While you might not be able to control your child's eye or hair color, you do have a great deal of influence on whether or not they are intelligent, compassionate, and kind, regardless of the origin of their chromosomes.

Okay, let's now get back to your options. We'll tackle them one by one.

∾ Sperm Donation ∾

Sperm donation is typically employed when a man has no viable sperm (azoospermia), even after corrective surgery or testicular biopsy, or if sperm quality has proven to be extremely poor over numerous cycles and is projected to be the couple's primary cause of infertility. Sperm donation is also commonly used when same-sex female couples choose to have a child or when a woman chooses to have a child on her own. Cryo-banks house frozen sperm and contain catalogs of prospective matches, offering couples (or singles) detailed information on family history, educational background, and physical attributes.

∾ Egg Donation ∾

This fairly new technology is starting to become more common, especially among women of advanced maternal age who have exhausted their chances of becoming pregnant using their own ova. Choosing to use an egg donor is more complicated than using a sperm donor because a donor is selected and typically goes through an IVF cycle while the recipient prepares to receive the embryos once they are at the blastocyst stage. This means choosing a donor from an agency, making sure she passes medical clearances, syncing up cycles with the intended mother, and progressing from there.

The cost of using an egg donor is roughly twice that of an IVF cycle, with at least half of that cost going to the donor herself and the agency representing her. Because prospective egg donors are in their prime reproductive years and have been screened for reproductive health, the chance of success on the first transfer is 60 to 70 percent. What's more, it is often the case that a donor cycle will result in leftover blastocysts, which can be frozen for future use.

For a woman over the age of 40 struggling with fertility due to egg quality, these odds are exponentially greater than her own. That said, there are still no guarantees. To hedge your bets, consider choosing a donor who has been successful donating in the past. The agency should be able to verify whether her previous cycles have resulted in pregnancies and live births.

Frozen egg banks are also cropping up around the United States. These banks offer ova that have already been harvested and frozen. While the price tag for each "lot" can be quite hefty, it is less expensive and can be less stressful than doing a "fresh" cycle. If you plan to have multiple kids and want them to be full biological siblings, this may not be the route for you, as the ova you purchased for baby number one might be all gone when you're ready for baby number two.

∽ Surrogacy ∽

Surrogates, also called gestational carriers, are women who offer (usually for a substantial fee) to carry a pregnancy for a woman whose uterus will not support a pregnancy. This can be the case for women whose mothers took a drug called DES (doctors mistakenly believed it would *prevent* pregnancy complications and losses), which caused uterine abnormalities and infertility in their offspring. Rarely, a woman is born without a uterus at all or may have a bicornuate uterus that is incompatible with pregnancy. Other uterine complications, such as immunologic infertility, cancer, excess scar tissue, or other deformities can preclude a woman from safely carrying a baby to term.

In some cases, surrogates also donate their ova to the couple in addition to carrying the baby. This practice is much less common, and in some states is illegal, as it is fraught with challenges should the gestational carrier (also the biological mother) have second thoughts. With donor ova becoming increasingly more common and accessible, couples faced with the inability to use the female's uterus or ova will often choose an egg donor and a separate gestational carrier.

In our practices, we often hear women confuse their diminished ovarian reserve or flagging egg quality with the need for a gestational carrier. It is important to remember that these two issues are mutually exclusive, with the need for surrogacy being much less common than the need for donor ova.

～ Adoption ～

Choosing to switch gears from producing your own offspring to adopting a child can prove to be a very difficult and complex decision.

People who are not faced with this decision often don't realize that we humans only have two biological imperatives: to survive and to procreate. For some couples, making the switch to adoption is smooth and easy; for some it's even a first choice. For others, the switch is painful, and they may feel resistant or even resentful about letting go of their dream of having a biological child.

One thing that seems universal is that once an adoptive family has that new baby or child in their arms, the resentment, fear, and anguish slowly (or quickly) melts away. The bonds of parenthood far outweigh the biological imperative, and the new family finds their way to the same kind of connections biological families have. Of course there can be complicating factors with adoption, which are outside the scope of this book. Still, for most, the upsides far outweigh the down.

In the United States, there are a few types of adoption to consider:

✳ **PRIVATE ADOPTION:** This process typically entails finding an adoption lawyer and creating a profile about yourself and your partner, which can be seen by women/ parents considering giving up a child for adoption. At some point, the prospective family is chosen or "matched" with a woman, and if all goes well, the baby is adopted by them, at or around the time of its birth. The potential downside to this type of adoption is that each state has a grace period, anywhere from 48 hours to one year, wherein the birth mother can change her mind and choose to keep the child.

✳ **INTERNATIONAL ADOPTION:** This process involves enlisting at an adoption agency and filing a petition with the country you want to adopt from. The adoptions are finalized either in the United States or abroad, depending on the rules for that particular country. Most of the children adopted from overseas have been placed in orphanages prior to being matched.

✳ **FOSTER CARE:** This form of adoption entails taking children who are wards of the state into your home. Some children are up for adoption, others are in limbo while waiting to see if they can return to their parent(s). Fostering to adopt can be extremely gratifying and is the least costly of all the adoption options.

Conclusion

We know how overwhelming it can be to make big lifestyle changes. The truth is, we've been there, too. We weren't born into families that emphasized nutrition, low stress, healthy living . . . we arrived there after years of our own unique struggles and explorations. And we're not perfect, either. We have our days when we're not inspired to cook, or when stress gets the better of us, ruining a night's sleep and sabotaging the next morning's workout. Still, we persevere.

What's our best advice for implementing choices that will "feed" every aspect of your life? Take it one bite at a time. Rather than turning your world upside down, start slowly and intentionally. Here are a few ideas for using this book efficiently, without adding more stress to your life:

- **Review the Cheat Sheet for Feeding Your Fertility (page 124) and the sections on conscious conception, self-care, and building a support team (pages 33-44).** Note the things you are doing already. You might just be surprised.
- **Make a list of the things that you think will be *easy* to implement and try adding a few of those things each week.** Maybe you'll start adding organic produce, raw milk, or grass-fed beef onto your weekly shopping list. Or get back into your favorite exercise or try a meditation CD before bed.
- **Make a list of the things that you imagine will be *hard* to implement and try adding one of those per week.** Maybe try a daily 10-minute meditation, a brisk morning walk, or even some spaghetti sauce made with a touch of "hidden" liver?
- **Follow the principle "slow and steady wins the race."** We've all been down the road of crash diets, exercise fads, and self-help phenomena. Much of the time, these things take us to extremes which can be fun and exhilarating at first, but ultimately end up being unsustainable. What we are proposing in this book is a lifestyle, not a fad, and we hope you'll find a way to make it your own and make it last.
- **Try a week of real food.** We've put together a week's meal plan on page 211.
- **Get support.** We are here to help. If you live in Los Angeles, we'd be happy to work with you in person. If you don't, we offer phone consultations. You can also pursue finding a practitioner in your area who is familiar with these principles and who knows about holistic and integrative fertility care.

It is our sincerest hope that you will find your way to optimal wellness in body, mind, and spirit, and that from that place of balance and health, you will cultivate true fertility in all aspects of your life.

Appendix

· ·

We've laid out a week's worth of meals below so you can get a feel for how to fit in your fertility foods with ease.

SUNDAY
Breakfast: Sourdough or sprouted toast with avocado and a fresh seasonal fruit salad
Lunch: Bacon Tomato Quiche with Cauliflower Crust (page 94)
Dinner: Basic Roast Chicken and Root Veggie Purée (page 101) and a simple salad

MONDAY
Breakfast: Thick strained yogurt with fresh berries and raw honey
Lunch: Bacon Tomato Quiche with Cauliflower Crust (page 94)
Dinner: Slow Cooker Beef and Mushroom Stew (page 80)

TUESDAY
Breakfast: Mini-Frittatas (page 93) and Creamy Delight Smoothie (page 77)
Lunch: Leftover Slow Cooker Beef and Mushroom Stew (page 80)
Dinner: Monica's Chicken Liver Pâté (page 99) and raw cheese on crackers

WEDNESDAY
Breakfast: Creamy Egg Drop Soup (page 95)
Lunch: Monica's Chicken Liver Pâté (page 99) and raw cheese on crackers
Dinner: Simple Veggie Soup (page 107) with homemade chicken stock (made from Sunday's chicken bones)

THURSDAY
Breakfast: Hard-boiled eggs and sourdough or sprouted toast with butter
Lunch: Leftover Simple Veggie Soup (page 107)
Dinner: Mustard-Crusted Salmon (page 114) and Wilted Dandelion Greens with Lemon and Feta (page 117)

FRIDAY
Breakfast: Green Soup (page 116) with leftover Mustard-Crusted Salmon (page 114)
Lunch: Green salad with hardboiled eggs and Ranch Dressing (page 76)
Dinner: California Burgers (page 97)

SATURDAY
Breakfast: Bacon and eggs with a side of sauerkraut
Lunch: Ceviche and Coconut Oil Tortilla Chips (page 112)
Dinner: Eat out and relax! (Order oysters, pâté, or bone marrow if it's on the menu!)

～ Glossary of Medical Terms ～

AMH (ANTI-MÜLLERIAN HORMONE): In women, AMH is a hormone secreted by the granulosa cells in the ovary. AMH levels predict ovarian reserve and decline with age.

ART (ASSISTED REPRODUCTIVE TECHNOLOGIES): This is a term used to describe methods of achieving pregnancy by artificial or partially artificial means, including IVF, IUI, and ICSI.

D&C (DILATION AND CURETTAGE): This is a surgical procedure wherein the cervix is dilated and the uterine lining is scraped with a tool called a curette. This performed in the case of missed miscarriage, abortion, or other uterine conditions.

E2 (ESTRADIOL): A female steroid hormone produced by the mature ovarian follicles and the adrenal cortex, it prepares the uterine lining for implantation and plays a significant role in maintaining reproductive health. It is used synthetically in ART.

FSH (FOLLICLE STIMULATING HORMONE): This is a hormone produced by the pituitary gland that signals the ovary to develop a follicle. Numbers tend to climb as we age because the ovaries' ability to produce estrogen declines.

GNRH (GONADOTROPIN RELEASING HORMONE): This is a hormone produced by the hypothalamus, which signals the anterior pituitary to secrete LH and FSH. It is also referred to as luteinizing hormone-releasing hormone.

HSG (HYSTEROSALPINGOGRAM): This is a radiologic procedure used to visualize the shape of the uterine cavity and to check for tubal patency.

ICSI (INTRACYTOPLASMIC SPERM INJECTION): This is a laboratory procedure wherein a single sperm is injected directly into an egg, for the purpose of overcoming male infertility.

IUI (INTRAUTERINE INSEMINATION): This is a procedure wherein sperm is deposited into the uterus via a fine tube (catheter) threaded through the cervix.

IVF (IN VITRO FERTILIZATION): This is a procedure wherein a woman's ovaries are stimulated to produce multiple mature eggs, followed by their removal. Once removed, they are fertilized in a laboratory and returned to the uterus three to five days later as embryos.

LH (LUTENEIZING HORMONE A.K.A. LUTROPIN OR LUTROPHIN): This is a hormone produced by the anterior pituitary. In women, an acute rise in LH (the LH surge) triggers ovulation and the development of the corpus luteum. In men, it stimulates the production of testosterone.

OB-GYN (OBSTETRICIAN-GYNECOLOGIST): This is a doctor who specializes in delivering babies and in the treatment of female gynecological conditions, including surgical procedures.

P4 (PROGESTERONE): This is a hormone secreted by the corpus luteum during the luteal phase that stimulates the uterine lining to prepare for pregnancy.

PRL (PROLACTIN): This is a hormone released by the anterior pituitary gland that stimulates the production of milk following childbirth.

RE (REPRODUCTIVE ENDOCRINOLOGIST): This is a surgical subspecialty of obstetrics and gynecology. Where physicians are trained to evaluate and treat hormone function as it pertains to reproduction and infertility.

TSH (THYROID STIMULATING HORMONE): This is a hormone secreted by the pituitary gland, which controls the release of T4 by the thyroid.

∼ References ∽

Allbritton, Jen. 2010. "Sacred Foods for Exceptionally Healthy Babies . . . and Parents, Too!" Weston A. Price Foundation. Accessed July 24, 2013. www.westonaprice.org/health-topics/sacred-foods-for-exceptionally-healthy-babies-and-parents-too.

American Society for Reproductive Medicine. 2012. "Age and Fertility." Accessed July 24, 2013. www.asrm.org/uploadedFiles/ASRM_Content/Resources/Patient_Resources/Fact_Sheets_and_Info_Booklets/agefertility.pdf.

Anthony, Mark. 2012. "Is Algae DHA as Healthy as Fish Oil DHA?" *Food Processing.* Accessed July 24, 2013. www.foodprocessing.com/articles/2012/algae-dha-healthy-as-fish-oil/.

Attia, Peter. 2012. "Ketosis—Advantaged or Misunderstood State? (Part I)." *The Eating Academy* (blog). Accessed July 24, 2013. http://eatingacademy.com/nutrition/ketosis-advantaged-or-misunderstood-state-part-i.

Bernardi, Lia A., and Mary Ellen Pavone. 2013. "Endometriosis." *Women's Health.* 2013;9(3):233–250. Accessed July 24, 2013. www.medscape.com/viewarticle/803830_3.

Carroll, N., and J. R. Palmer. "A Comparison of Intrauterine Versus Intracervical Insemination in Fertile Single Women." *Fertility and Sterility.* Apr;200175(4):656–60 [Abstract]. Accessed July 24, 2013. www.ncbi.nlm.nih.gov/pubmed/11287014.

Chavarro, J. E., et al. "A Prospective Study of Dairy Foods Intake and Anovulatory Infertility." *Oxford Journals, Human Reproduction.* 2007;22(5):1340–47. Accessed July 24, 2013. http://humrep.oxfordjournals.org/content/22/5/1340.full.

Daniel, Kaayla T. 2003. "Why Broth Is Beautiful: Essential Roles for Proline, Glycine and Gelatin." Weston A. Price Foundation. Accessed July 24, 2013. www.westonaprice.org/food-features/why-broth-is-beautiful.

Danielsson, Krissi. 2009. "Bacterial and Viral Infections Linked to Miscarriage/Pregnancy Loss." Accessed July 24, 2013. http://miscarriage.about.com/od/infections/tp/infections.htm.

De Lacey, Sheryl, et al. 2009. "Building Resilience: A Preliminary Exploration of Women's Perceptions of the Use of Acupuncture as an Adjunct to In Vitro Fertilisation." BMC Complementary and Alternative Medicine. Accessed July 24, 2013. www.biomedcentral.com/1472-6882/9/50.

European Commission. n.d. "Rules on GMOs in the EU—Ban on GMOs." Accessed July 24, 2013. http://ec.europa.eu/food/food/biotechnology/gmo_ban_cultivation_en.htm.

Fallon, Sally, and Mary Enig. 2002. "Vitamin A Saga." Weston A. Price Foundation. Accessed July 24, 2013. www.westonaprice.org/fat-soluble-activators/vitamin-a-saga.

Flower, A., et al. 2012. "Chinese Herbal Medicine for Endometriosis." *Cochrane Database of Systematic Reviews.* May 16;5:CD006568 [Abstract]. Accessed July 24, 2013. www.ncbi.nlm.nih.gov/pubmed/22592712.

Gerster, H. 1998. "Can Adults Adequately Convert Alpha-Linolenic Acid (18:3n-3) to Eicosapentaenoic Acid (20:5n-3) and Docosahexaenoic Acid (22:6n-3)?" *International Journal for Vitamin and Nutrition Research.* 1998;68(3):159-73 [Abstract]. Accessed July 24, 2013. www.ncbi.nlm.nih.gov/pubmed/9637947#.

Gibiru, Kaiser. 2012. "Permanente Comes Out Against GMO." *Gibiru Uncensored News.* Accessed July 24, 2013. http://gibiru.com/index.php/uncensored-news/78-news/25456-kaiser-permanente-comes-out-against-gmo.

Green America. 2012. "Who Requires Labels?" Accessed July 24, 2013. www.greenamerica.org/pubs/greenamerican/articles/AprilMay2012/Who-requires-GMO-labels.cfm.

Harvard Health Publications. 2009. "The Psychological Impact of Infertility and Its Treatment." Accessed July 24, 2013. www.health.harvard.edu/newsletters/Harvard_Mental_Health_Letter/2009/May.

Hoag, S. W. 1997. "Failure of Prescription Prenatal Vitamin Products to Meet USP Standards for Folic Acid Dissolution." *American Journal of the Pharmacology Association,* July–August, 1997.

Hollis, B. W., et al. 2011. "Vitamin D Supplementation During Pregnancy: Double-Blind, Randomized Clinical Trial of Safety and Effectiveness." *J Bone Miner Res.* 2011 Oct;26(10):2341–57. Accessed July 24, 2013. www.ncbi.nlm.nih.gov/pubmed/21706518.

Hullender, Rubin L., M. S. Opsahl, K. Wiemer, et al. "The Effects of Adjuvant Whole-systems Traditional Chinese Medicine on In Vitro Fertilization Live Births: A Retrospective Cohort Study." [Abstract] *J Alt Complement Med.* 2014;20(5):A12–A13.

Human Genome Project. n.d. "The Science Behind the Human Genome Project: Understanding the Basics." Accessed July 24, 2013. http://web.ornl.gov/sci/techresources/Human_Genome/project/info.shtml.

Institute for Responsible Technology. n.d. "Genetically Modified Soy Linked to Sterility, Infant Mortality." Accessed July 24, 2013. www.responsibletechnology.org/article-gmo-soy-linked-to-sterility.

IVF Worldwide. n.d. "Age Related Infertility." Accessed July 24, 2013. www.ivfworldwide.com/education/patients-investigation-and-evaluation/age-related-infertility.html.

Janevic, Teresa, et al. 2014. "Effects of Work and Life Stress on Semen Quality." *Fertility and Sterility.* doi:10.1016/j.fertnstert.2014.04.021.

Jensen, T. K., et al. 2013. "Association of Sleep Disturbances with Reduced Semen Quality: A Cross-Sectional Study Among 953 Healthy Young Danish Men." *American Journal of Epidemiology,* 2013. 177(10):1027–37.

Labyak, S., et al. 2002. "Effects of Shiftwork on Sleep and Menstrual Function in Nurses." *Health Care for Women International.* Sep–Nov 2002;23(6–7):703–14 [Abstract]. Accessed July 24, 2013. www.ncbi.nlm.nih.gov/pubmed/12418990.

Leproult R., and E. Van Cauter. 2011. "Effect of 1 Week of Sleep Restriction on Testosterone Levels in Young Healthy Men." *Journal of the American Medical Association,* 2011. 305(21):2173–4. Accessed July 24, 2013. http://jama.jamanetwork.com/article.aspx?articleid=1029127.

Lerchbaum, E., and B. Obermayer-Pietsch. 2012. "Vitamin D and Fertility: A Systematic Review." *European Journal of Endocrinology,* 2012 May;166(5):765–78 [Abstract]. Accessed July 24, 2013. www.ncbi.nlm.nih.gov/pubmed/22275473.

Lewis, Randine. 2004. *Infertility Cure: The Ancient Chinese Wellness Program for Getting Pregnant and Having Healthy Babies.* New York, NY: Little, Brown and Company.

Lima, A. P., et al. 2006. "Prolactin and Cortisol Levels in Women with Endometriosis." *Brazilian Journal of Medical and Biological Research*. 2006; 39(8):1121–7 [Abstract]. Accessed July 24, 2013. www.ncbi.nlm.nih.gov/pubmed/16906287.

Lynch, C.D., et al. 2014. "Preconception stress increases the risk of infertility: results from a couple-based prospective cohort study—the LIFE study." *Human Reproduction*. 2014; 29(5): 1067–75.

Mancini, A., and G. Balercia. 2011. "Coenzyme Q(10) in Male Infertility: Physiopathology and Therapy." *Biofactors*. 2011 Sep–Oct;37(5):374–80 [Abstract]. Accessed July 24, 2013. www.ncbi.nlm.nih.gov/pubmed/21989906.

Mancini, A., et al. 2005. "An Update of Coenzyme Q10 Implications in Male Infertility: Biochemical and Therapeutic Aspects." *Biofactors*. 2005;25(1-4):165–74 [Abstract]. Accessed July 24, 2013. www.ncbi.nlm.nih.gov/pubmed/16873942.

Manheimer, E., et al. 2005. "Effects of Acupuncture on Rates of Pregnancy and Live Birth among Women Undergoing In Vitro Fertilisation: Systematic Review and Meta-analysis." *British Medical Journal*, 2008;336:545. [Abstract]. Accessed June 2, 2014. www.bmj.com/content/336/7643/545.

Masterjohn, Chris. 2008. "On the Trail of the Elusive X-Factor: A Sixty-Two-Year-Old Mystery Finally Solved." Weston A. Price Foundation. Accessed July 24, 2013. www.westonaprice.org/fat-soluble-activators/x-factor-is-vitamin-k2#fig4.

Mendonça, L. L. F., et al. 2000. "Non-Steroidal Anti-Inflammatory Drugs as a Possible Cause for Reversible Infertility." *Rheumatology*, 2000. 39(8):880–82 [Abstract]. Accessed July 24, 2013. www.ncbi.nlm.nih.gov/pubmed/10952743.

Meyer, Hartmut. n.d. "Effects of Roundup on Mammalian Fertility." *Third World Network*. Accessed July 24, 2013. http://twnside.org.sg/title/effec-cn.htm.

Michaelis, Kristin. 2013. Beautiful Babies: Nutrition for Fertility, Pregnancy, Breast-feeding, and Baby's First Foods. Auberry, CA: Victory Belt Publishing.

Nagel, Ramiel. 2009. Cure Tooth Decay: Heal and Prevent Cavities with Nutrition. Ashland, OR: Golden Child.

Paulus, Wolfgang. 2002. "Influence of Acupuncture on the Pregnancy Rate in Patients Who Undergo Assisted Reproduction Therapy." *Fertility and Sterility*, April 2002. 77(4):721–24 [Abstract]. Accessed July 24, 2013. www.fertstert.org/article/S0015-0282(01)03273-3/abstract.

Phys.org. 2005. "Study: High Mortality Rats Ate GM Food." Accessed July 24, 2013. http://phys.org/news7740.html.

Planck, Nina. 2006. Real Food: What to Eat and Why. New York, NY: Bloomsbury.

Pollan, Michael. 2008. In Defense of Food : An Eater's Manifesto. New York, NY: Penguin.

Porter, Robert, ed. 2011. *Merck Manual of Diagnosis and Therapy 19th Edition*. White House Station, NJ: Merck Sharpe & Dohme Corp.

Price, Weston. 1989. *Nutrition and Physical Degeneration*. La Mesa, CA: Price-Pottenger Nutrition Foundation.

Razaitis, Lynn. 2005. "The Liver Files." Weston A. Price Foundation. Accessed July 24, 2013. www.westonaprice.org/food-features/liver-files.

Ross, Julia. 1999. *The Diet Cure: The 8-Step Program to Rebalance Your Body Chemistry and End Food Cravings, Weight Gain, and Mood Swings—Naturally*. New York, NY: Penguin.

Salatin, Joel. 2011. Folks, This Ain't Normal. New York, NY: Center Street Hachette Book Group.

Smith-Spangler, Crystal, et al. 2012. "Are Organic Foods Safer or Healthier than Conventional Alternatives?: A Systematic Review." *Annals of Internal Medicine*. September 2012;157(5). Accessed July 24, 2013. http://annals.org/article.aspx?articleid=1355685.

Steiner-Victorin, Elisabet, et al. 1996. "Reduction of Blood Flow Impedance in the Uterine Arteries of Infertile Women with Electro-Acupuncture." *Human Reproduction,* 1996 June;11(6):1314–7. Accessed July 24, 2013. http://yourivfacupuncture.com/what-is-the-process/research/medical-research-article-1.

Udoff, Laurence, and Grant Zhang. 2010. "The Impact of Complementary Medicine on In Vitro Fertilization." *Reproductive Endocrinology and Infertility*. 2010:727–37 [Abstract]. Accessed July 24, 2013. http://link.springer.com/chapter/10.1007/978-1-4419-1436-1_50.

U.S. Department of Agriculture. 2004. "Nutrient Content of the U.S. Food Supply, 1909-2000." Home Economics Research Report No. 56. Accessed July 24, 2013. www.cnpp.usda.gov/publications/foodsupply/foodsupply1909-2000.pdf.

Vitamin D Council. n.d. "How Do I Get the Vitamin D My Body Needs?" Accessed July 24, 2013. www.vitamindcouncil.org/about-vitamin-d/how-do-i-get-the-vitamin-d-my-body-needs.

Acknowedgments

FROM EMILY

Thanks to everyone who has helped with the birth and evolution of this book. To my husband/provider/proofreader/kitchen-cleaner/kid-entertainer for being the awesome partner that you are—I am so grateful for this wild journey we are braving together. To my two beautiful children for dealing with "busy-cranky mom" after long days of writing and editing and for always being my mirror, reminding me when it's time to slow down and appreciate this beautiful life. To Monica Ford for the inspiration for many of the delicious recipes included in this book. To my mentor, Yvonne Farrell, for encouraging and guiding me to my true potential as a practitioner. And to Laura Erlich, for bringing your fantastic nerdy knowledge, dedication, and humor—you've made this project super fun, and I couldn't imagine a better writing partner.

FROM LAURA

First thanks go to my writing partner, Emily Bartlett—your motivation, depth of knowledge, and fun energy have made this process a true joy. Still, I couldn't have done my part without the unwavering support of my super-dad husband Sean, the most kind and loving partner I could ever have dreamed up. To my partner in business and crime, Trace Albrecht, and my dear friend and mentor, Yvonne Farrell, I'd be utterly lost without you both. A huge thanks to Dr. Kelly Baek, for your generous time in editing the ART sections and for always being a phone call away, both personally and professionally. Deep gratitude to the awesome women of my profession, most notably Randine Lewis, Jill Blakeway, and Lee Hullender-Rubin for being genuinely helpful and supportive. Special thanks to Ray Rubio for making me your grasshopper, and to Lorne Brown for getting behind this book in its early stages.

To my amazing son, Sebastian—you are the light of my life and I will always love you more! And to my wonderful family and friends, especially my sister Nina, aunt Dorien, and stepdaughter Erin for being my steadfast and loving support system. Lastly, to the memory of my mom and dad, Heidi and Harvey—even in your absence, I strive to do you proud.

And, of course—thank YOU, our reader, for your bravery along this journey to parenthood and for entrusting us to be your guides to cultivating fertility every step of the way.

About the Authors

EMILY BARTLETT, LAC runs a Chinese medicine practice in Los Angeles, California. When she's not seeing patients or hanging at the beach with her husband and two lively kids, you can find her blog at HolisticSquid.com about fertility, natural health, and nutrition.

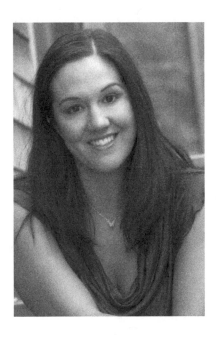

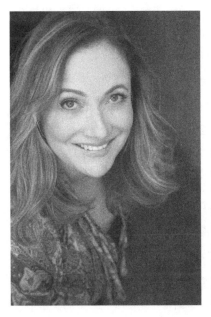

LAURA ERLICH, LAC (FABORM) is the co-clinic director of LA Herbs and Acupuncture, in West Los Angeles, California. In addition to her clinical practice, she teaches continuing education classes to other acupuncturists and attends births as a doula. You can find more of her writings on her blog, ABaoInTheOven.com. She is luckier than lucky to share her life with her wonderful husband, hilarious son, and beautiful stepdaughter.

Recipe Index

General Index

pH balance and, 27
Qi and, 186
risk factors, 184–185
"Rob," 187
semen analysis, 185–186
sleep and, 39
stress and, 9
vitamins and, 187
Western medicine and, 184–185
Spleen/Stomach system, 49, 62–63, 66–68
stimulated IUI (intrauterine insemination), 195
stress
    allostasis, 35
    conception attempts and, 9
    fight-or-flight response, 9, 34
    hormones and, 39
    managing, 34–35
    nervous system and, 9
    sleep and, 39
    sperm and, 9
    unexplained infertility and, 181
support teams
    Chinese medicine, 42–43
    group therapy, 42
    individual therapy, 42
    medical support, 43, 44
    OB-GYNs (obstetrician-gynecologists), 44
    Resolve organization, 42
    support groups, 41–42
    therapy, 42
surrogacy, 208

tai qi, 38
tea, 118
teeth, 58–60
therapy, 42
thyroid issues
    communication and, 177
    diet and lifestyle and, 178
    Hashimoto's thyroiditis, 175, 177
    hyperthyroidism, 176, 177
    hypothyroidism, 174–175, 176
    "Jill," 179
toxins
    clearing, 70
    filters for, 11
    GMOs (genetically-modified organisms) and, 20
    medications, 12–14
    pesticides, 16–17, 20
    water and, 10, 11
    xenoestrogens, 10–11
trace minerals, 144
TSH (Thyroid Stimulating Hormone), 191

ultrasounds, 193
unexplained infertility
    Chinese medicine and, 180–182
    "Marni," 183
    reproductive energy and, 182
    stress and, 181
    Western medicine and, 180

vegetables, 128–129

vegetarianism, 121–123
vitamins
    B-complex, 142–143
    calcium, 127
    choline, 127
    cod liver oil, 131–132, 135, 136
    folic acid, 127
    iron, 127
    IVF (in vitro fertilization) and, 203
    krill oil, 132–133
    multivitamins, 136, 150
    omega-3s, 127, 131–133
    prenatal vitamins, 150
    raw milk and, 81
    saturated fats and, 74
    seafood, 110
    sperm and, 187
    vegetarianism and, 121, 122–123
    vitamin A, 128, 137–138
    vitamin B_6, 127, 142
    vitamin B_{12}, 127, 143
    vitamin C, 145–146
    vitamin D, 127, 134–136
    vitamin D_3, 135–136
    vitamin K_2, 138–140
    zinc, 127

water
    filtering, 11
    recommendations, 119
    xenoestrogens and, 10
Western medicine
    acupuncture and, 42–43
    age, 152–153
    Chinese medicine and, 54–56
    endometriosis and, 160–161
    foods and, 57–58
    hyperthyroidism, 176
    miscarriage and, 156, 158
    OB-GYNs (obstetrician-gynecologists), 44
    PCOS (Polycystic Ovary Syndrome) and, 170–171
    seeking, 43
    sperm and, 184–185
    unexplained infertility and, 180
whole grains. See grains.

xenoestrogens, 10–11, 68, 163

Yin and Yang, 45–46, 61, 69–70
yoga, 37–38

zinc, 127